Osteoarthritis

YOUR QUESTIONS ANSWERED

D0531179

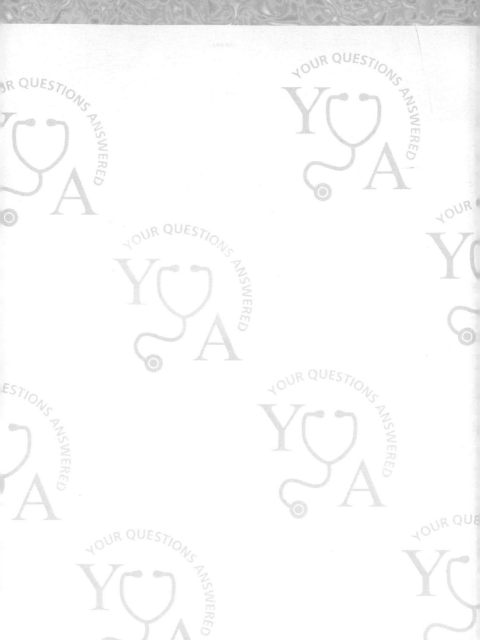

Commissioning and development: Fiona Conn
Project Manager: Frances Affleck
Design direction: George Ajayi
Illustrator: Ethan Danielson

Osteoarthritis

YOUR QUESTIONS ANSWERED

John Dickson
MB ChB, MRCGP, FRCP (London), FRCP (Glasgow)
Primary Care Rheumatologist; Co-founder, Primary Care Rheumatology Society

Gillian Hosie
MB ChB, FRCP (Glasgow), DA
General Practitioner, Glasgow, UK; Past President, Primary Care Rheumatology
Society

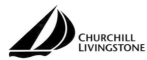

EDINBURGH LONDON NEW YORK OXFORD PHILADELPHIA ST LOUIS SYDNEY TORONTO 2003

CHURCHILL LIVINGSTONE
An imprint of Elsevier Science Limited

First published 2003

ISBN 0 443 07346 5

British Library Cataloguing in Publication Data
A catalogue record for this book is available from the British Library

Library of Congress Cataloging in Publication Data
A catalog record for this book is available from the Library of Congress

Notice
Medical knowledge is constantly changing. Standard safety precautions must be followed,
but as new research and clinical experience broaden our knowledge, changes in treatment
and drug therapy may become necessary or appropriate. Readers are advised to check the
most current product information provided by the manufacturer of each drug to be
administered to verify the recommended dose, the method and duration of administration,
and contraindications. It is the responsibility of the practitioner, relying on experience and
knowledge of the patient, to determine dosages and the best treatment for each individual
patient. Neither the Publisher nor the author/editor/contributor (*delete as appropriate*)
assumes any liability for any injury and/or damage to persons or property arising from this
publication.

your source for books,
journals and multimedia
in the health sciences
www.elsevierhealth.com

The
publisher's
policy is to use
paper manufactured
from sustainable forests

Printed in China

Contents

Preface

Osteoarthritis is a very common condition that affects a huge number of people, mostly in the older age groups. It causes enormous demands on health care providers, carers and society at large, as well as reducing the quality of life for many people due to pain and disability. As well as the social costs, the financial costs of the condition are also extremely high, with very large sums being spent on drug therapy and joint replacements. As the population ages and with increased life-expectancy, the burden of osteoarthritis will continue to rise and place increasing demands on an already stretched health service.

Traditionally, doctors have found the management of osteoarthritis dull, difficult and uninspiring and have tended to accord it a low profile. There are a number of reasons for this: there is no cure for osteoarthritis; osteoarthritis has been regarded as an almost inevitable consequence of growing older; drug therapy is often associated with major side-effects and joint replacements were undertaken when patients were in end-stage osteoarthritis and often too frail and unfit to benefit fully from their surgery.

Increasingly, research has suggested that osteoarthritis is a dynamic rather than a purely degenerative condition and that physical therapies and lifestyle changes can have considerable impact on a patient's quality of life. This has resulted in a much more holistic attitude to the management of osteoarthritis, with patients themselves becoming more involved in managing their own condition.

This book considers all aspects of the condition of osteoarthritis from pathophysiology and epidemiology through diagnosis and joint examination. Methods of managing osteoarthritis are discussed in detail, with particular emphasis on non-pharmacological therapies. As drug therapy will be required by most patients at some time in the course of the disease, topical, oral and injection therapies are all reviewed with up-to-date information on new therapies.

Most patients with osteoarthritis can be managed within primary care, and this book should provide the practical tools to help primary care providers achieve this aim. Inevitably though, some patients will require referral, and the chapters on referral and surgical options provide guidance as to when referral is appropriate. Long-term outlook is discussed in the chapter on prognosis.

Following many of the chapters there is a section on frequently asked questions. These are useful not only for patients with osteoarthritis and their friends and carers but also for members of the primary care team.

Osteoarthritis is moving on from being a 'cinderella' subject and is now the topic of much research into the development of new drugs designed not only to treat the condition but also to prevent its development. Lifestyle changes such as weight loss and increased exercise fit well with prevention programmes for other chronic diseases such as coronary heart disease, diabetes and osteoporosis.

This book provides practical and pragmatic advice about the management of osteoarthritis and should act as a resource for all members of the primary care team.

JD
GH

How to use this book

The *Your Questions Answered* series aims to meet the information needs of GPs and other primary care professionals who care for patients with chronic conditions. It is designed to help them work with patients and their families, providing effective, evidence-based care and management.

The books are in an accessible question and answer format, with detailed contents lists at the beginning of every chapter and a complete index to help find specific information.

ICONS
Icons are used in the book to identify particular types of information:

 highlights important information

 highlights side-effect information.

PATIENT QUESTIONS
At the end of relevant chapters there are sections of frequently asked patient questions, with easy-to-understand answers aimed at the non-medical reader. These questions are also listed at the end of the book.

Aetiology, epidemiology and pathophysiology of osteoarthritis

1

1.1 How common is OA?

OA is the commonest disorder of joints. It is more common in older age groups and causes considerable problems with disability and pain in the elderly. The knee is the commonest large joint affected by OA, with hip the next commonest. OA of these two joints affects around 10–25% of the population in those aged over 65. It is always difficult to get accurate figures for the prevalence of OA in the community as the results depend on whether inclusion is based on radiographic findings or clinical signs and symptoms. For example, the Framingham Study (Felson et al 1987) suggested that radiographic knee OA occurred in 33% of those aged over 63 whereas symptomatic knee OA was present in around 9.5%. Another study (Engel 1968) looked at radiographic hand OA and found a prevalence of 5% in adults aged under 35 and over 70% in those aged over 65. Peat et al (2001) estimated the prevalence of knee pain in an elderly population (see Box 1.1). Whatever the exact numbers, it is safe to say that the pain and disability of OA affects a large proportion of older patients.

1.2 Is OA more common in women than in men?

Below the age of 50, OA is more common in men but becomes more common in women over the age of 50 and this gender difference continues to increase with increasing age. It has been postulated that this age- and sex-related pattern may be associated with postmenopausal oestrogen deficiency. OA in women often has a more generalized distribution than in men, affecting many different joints.

1.3 Is OA more common in certain areas of the world or in certain ethnic groups?

Hip OA appears to be much less common in black and Asian populations than in Caucasians, although knee OA has been reported as being more

---

BOX 1.1 The prevalence of knee pain in an elderly population (based on data from Peat et al 2001)

In a primary care trust population of 100 000 aged over 55 years:
- 25 000 will have knee pain (4 weeks) in any year
- 4000 who consult their doctor with knee pain in any year will be diagnosed OA
- 1500 people with severely painful and disabling knee pain will be diagnosed OA.

common in black women than in white. The reasons for these apparent differences are not yet understood.

1.4 Do all elderly patients develop OA?

Symptomatic OA does not affect all of the older population and many elderly people remain free of any significant joint symptoms. If X-rays were taken of the joints of some of these patients it is probable that changes of OA would be present, but such findings are irrelevant if the patient is asymptomatic.

1.5 Is there a pattern of joint involvement in OA?

OA tends to affect certain joints and to spare others. Joints commonly affected are hip, knee, hand (in particular, the distal interphalangeal joints, the proximal interphalangeal joints and the carpometacarpal joint of the thumb), cervical spine, lumbosacral spine and the first metatarsophalangeal in the foot (*see Fig. 1.1*). Joints much less frequently affected are ankle, wrist, elbow and shoulder.

There are a number of common clinical patterns within the above groups (*see Box 1.2*).

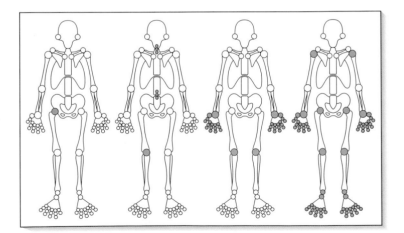

▲

Fig. 1.1 Four common clinical patterns of OA. From University of Bath Diploma in Primary Care Rheumatology 1995 with permission.

BOX 1.2 Common clinical patterns of OA

- Middle-aged to elderly woman with OA of hands and knee
- Middle-aged to older man with OA of one knee, often due to previous trauma
- Younger man with OA of one joint, usually hip, possibly due to dysplasia or to a genetic collagen abnormality
- Elderly woman with severe OA affecting several joints, including shoulders, hips and knees. The affected joints show large cool effusions containing apatite crystals. This is a painful progressive condition; when it occurs in the shoulder it is known as 'Milwaukee shoulder syndrome'

1.6 What are the causes of OA?

As research into OA progresses it is becoming clear that there is no one single cause of the condition. Genetic factors certainly have a place in the development of OA and it has been found that siblings of patients undergoing hip or knee replacements have a much higher risk of developing OA themselves—five times higher for hip OA and three times higher for knee OA (Doherty et al 2001). There is also a genetic component in 'nodal generalized OA'; for example, patients developing Heberden's nodes at the distal interphalangeal joints will often have a strong family history of similar nodes and indeed clinical OA. The development of Heberden's nodes act as a marker for the development of knee OA. Other factors may come into play in triggering OA in a genetically predisposed individual. These include trauma, mechanical factors and metabolic insults. It is thought that the condition of OA is the result of the joint trying to repair itself after these various insults and, although the joints are in a continual process of damage and repair, eventually, for a variety of reasons, the repair process can no longer keep up with the damage incurred and frank OA results.

1.7 Are there any risk factors for the development of OA?

A number of risk factors have been identified for the development of knee and hip OA (*see Box 1.3*).

BOX 1.3 Risk factors for the development of OA in knee and hip

For the knee these include:
- The presence of Heberden's nodes
- Female gender
- Increasing age
- Obesity
- Internal derangement and instability
- Occupations involving repetitive knee-bending
- Sports such as professional football.

For the hip these are:
- Caucasian race
- Increasing age (although less than for knee OA)
- Occupations such as farming
- Sports such as elite athletics
- Congenital and childhood hip disease, such as Perthe's disease, slipped femoral epiphysis, congenital dislocation of hip and forms of dysplasia.

1.8 Can any of these risk factors be modified to prevent the development of OA?

Obviously, factors such as genetic inheritance, increasing age and gender cannot be changed. Some of the other risk factors can certainly be modified and this should be considered in all patients with clinical OA as well as in those who are at risk.

Obesity is one risk factor that can be tackled. Studies have shown that not only does knee OA occur more commonly in the already overweight but that obesity precedes the development of knee OA. There is also an association of obesity with hip OA, although less strong than for knee OA and, perhaps surprisingly, obesity is also associated with an increase in hand OA. In the knee there is a considerable difference between the forces exerted across the knee joint in overweight subjects compared with those of normal weight. These differences do not apply to hand joints and therefore the association of obesity with hand OA remains puzzling. It may be that, in the overweight, there are other metabolic or hormonal factors not yet understood which are responsible for cartilage breakdown.

The long-term Framingham studies in the USA (Felson et al 1987) suggested that, in overweight subjects, weight loss significantly reduced the risk of developing symptomatic knee OA. Weight loss of 5 kg in women who had a body mass index of over 25 led to a 50% reduction in the risk of developing symptomatic knee OA (Felson et al 1992). There is also some evidence that, for patients who already have knee OA, weight reduction can reduce the rate of disease progression and can significantly reduce symptoms.

Various traumatic events can be risk factors for knee OA. These events, such as fracture, ligament damage or meniscal cartilage tears or previous knee surgery, probably cannot be prevented but some of the risks could possibly be reduced with improved training for sporting activities.

1.9   What are the childhood problems that can lead to the development of OA in later life?

These include Legg–Perthe's disease, congenital dislocation of the hip (CDH) and slipped femoral epiphysis. With increased childhood screening, hopefully most cases of CDH will be found and treated at an early age, thus reducing the long-term risk of hip OA. Most patients with Legg–Perthe's disease and slipped femoral epiphysis will eventually develop OA hip to some degree. This is because of changes resulting from abnormal loading around the joint.

Some patients are found to have a congenital condition of dysplasia at the hip. Dysplasia is really a mild form of CDH where the acetabulum is unusually shallow, resulting in abnormal biomechanics around the hip. It is thought that dysplasia may account for some of the hip OA seen in women, although probably not in men.

1.10   Are there any other pathologies that may predispose to OA?

Septic arthritis and avascular necrosis may lead to the later development of OA. Other conditions such as hypermobility (double-jointedness)—if the joint is allowed to overstretch—and unequal leg length again may lead to abnormal stresses around the joint and OA in later life.

1.11   If, as stated previously, postmenopausal oestrogen deficiency leads to the development of OA, does hormone replacement therapy (HRT) prevent this development?

Some recent studies looking at both symptomatic and radiographic disease have shown that HRT reduces the risk of both hip and knee OA. The benefit seems to be greater in those on long-term HRT (Hannan et al 1990, Nevitt et al 1994).

1.12 Is there any relationship between the development of OA and osteoporosis?

There appears to be a negative association between osteoporosis and OA, especially at the hip joint. It has been suggested that in patients who develop OA subchondral bone may be harder due to sclerosis, whereas in patients more likely to develop osteoporosis the bone may be softer and more readily deformable. Obesity, which predisposes to OA, tends to protect against osteoporosis. Interestingly, HRT should help to protect against both OA and osteoporosis.

1.13 Are there any particular jobs that are more likely to cause OA?

Certain occupations seem to predispose to the development of OA. These include: farmers whose job involves such activities as bending, lifting heavy weights and walking long distances over rough ground and who have a higher than average rate of hip OA; miners, whose job involves much bending often in cramped spaces and who have a higher incidence of knee and spine OA; and those working in jobs involving a lot of bending with the knee in a close-packed position, such as joiners and carpet layers, who have an increased incidence of knee OA.

Obviously it may not be possible to change an occupation in order to avoid developing OA. Many jobs such as farming involve many different activities and it may be difficult to identify the particular activity causing the problem. Economic factors also come into play here. Occupational physicians have a role to play in attempting to reduce unnecessary load-carrying, bending or other potential risk factors. This is particularly important in individuals who have a genetic tendency to develop OA.

1.14 Are there any particular sports that lead to the development of OA?

Football players certainly seem to have a higher than average rate of OA, but this seems to be related to the often major cartilage and ligament injuries sustained. Many of these players have had previous surgery to their knees, again increasing the risk.

Elite athletes seem to have a greater risk of lower limb OA. This seems to be related to the intensive and specialized training which they undergo, whereas there is at present no evidence that leisure running or jogging increases the risk of lower limb OA. Anecdotally, certain sports involving recurrent knee stress or injury (e.g. downhill ski-ing) or repeated trauma (e.g. parachuting) may lead to OA.

1.15 Is OA becoming more common?

There is no evidence that OA in itself is becoming more common. The population as a whole is living longer thus giving OA more chance to manifest itself; the impact of OA is therefore becoming a very serious health and social problem. The population as a whole is becoming more obese and more sedentary, again magnifying the problem.

1.16 What are the pathological changes in a joint with OA?

In the past, OA was thought of as a purely degenerative condition in which the articular cartilage inexorably broke down with increasing age. It is now recognized that OA is in fact a dynamic condition in which damage to the joint surfaces is balanced by a repair process. As time goes on, damage increases and eventually, despite an ever greater repair process, repair is unable to keep up with damage and the changes of OA occur (*see Fig. 1.2*).

The initial change is a breakdown of the articular cartilage in a small localized area. This leads to changes in the proteoglycan matrix, with increased activity of the chondrocytes and an increased water content. These changes reduce the impact-absorbing properties at this site, leading to the thinning and subsequent breakdown of the cartilage. At this stage, the repair process comes into play and attempts are made to increase vascularity and remodel the surface. Chondrocytes and osteophytes develop at the fibrocartilage edges of the joint areas, which potentially increases the joint area, possibly to help joint stability and possibly to increase the area available for articulation. At the same time changes occur in the surrounding bone. These include the development of areas of sclerosis as new bone develops to strengthen the existing trabecular structure and the development of bone cysts. Bone cysts develop because of raised intra-articular pressure in areas where the articular cartilage is missing. The increased pressure is transmitted to the marrow of the surrounding bone, resulting in these cysts, which may continue to enlarge until the pressure is equalized. At the same time, degradation products from bone and cartilage, possibly including apatite crystals, are deposited within the joint and may lead to an inflammatory type of reaction. This inflammation may produce areas of synovitis and eventually lead to effusion occurring within the joint. In the longer term, such effusions cause stretching of the joint capsule and eventual thickening.

1.17 How do the pathological changes of OA relate to the clinical picture of OA?

Pain, stiffness and functional impairment are the main symptoms of OA, and each symptom can be related to the pathological changes (*see Q. 1.16*) taking place within an OA joint.

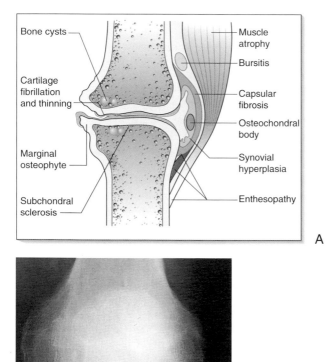

Bone cysts

Cartilage fibrillation and thinning

Marginal osteophyte

Subchondral sclerosis

Muscle atrophy

Bursitis

Capsular fibrosis

Osteochondral body

Synovial hyperplasia

Enthesopathy

A

B

Fig. 1.2 Diagram and X-ray of a knee showing early OA. From Kumar P, Clark M (eds) 2002 Clinical medicine, 5th edn (Saunders), with permission.

1.18 Are there any serum or urinary markers for OA?

At present there are no blood or urine tests that reflect either clinical OA or any predisposing factors. Where there is doubt about the diagnosis, blood tests are sometimes useful in order to exclude other conditions (*see Q. 2.14*).

1.19 Is OA a purely degenerative disease?

The phrase 'degenerative disease' suggests a condition in which tissues become inevitably broken down in a one-way process. As described above (*see Q. 1.16*), although there is breakdown of tissue in all joints there is accompanying regeneration and it is only when the breakdown exceeds repair that the changes of OA occur.

There does seem to be an inflammatory component in the changes that take place in a joint affected by OA. This low-grade inflammation is not reflected in changes in inflammatory markers such as raised erythrocyte sedimentation rate (ESR) or C-reactive protein (CRP). Inflammatory flares with increased pain and stiffness and sometimes signs of mild synovitis may occur during the course of chronic OA and are often related to unaccustomed overuse or mild trauma.

1.20 What is the function of the synovial fluid within a joint?

Synovial fluid is an important constituent of a synovial joint. Not only does it act as a lubricant and shock-absorber due to the hyaluronan present within it, but it also acts as a conduit for nutrients and may also, together with the synovial membrane, have messenger and hormonal functions. In a normal joint, the hyaluronan present is of high molecular weight and it is this particular property that is thought to contribute to its lubricating and shock-absorbing properties. Within joints there are pain-mediating receptors known as nociceptors, and high-molecular-weight hyaluronan found in a normal joint is thought to have a protective effect on these nociceptors. In a joint affected by OA, the hyaluronan has been found to be of a lower molecular weight. We do not yet know whether this lower-molecular-weight hyaluronan is produced in response to the pathological condition, or whether it is compensatory or indeed whether it is the initial factor in the whole pathological process. This lower-molecular-weight hyaluronan may have reduced ability to act as a shock-absorber and as a lubricant and may be less effective in protecting the nociceptors.

1.21 What are the main signs and symptoms of OA?

When a joint is affected by OA it tends to look enlarged compared with the normal. This is due to the bony changes of osteophyte growth at the joint margins. In progressively severe OA there may also be deformity, such as varus deformity at the knee or a fixed-flexion deformity at the hip. Joint line tenderness is often present and there may be some soft tissue tenderness from peri-articular structures such as the anserine bursa at the knee (*see Fig. 1.3*). There may be a small cool effusion present. Movement of the joint may show a decreased range of movement and often coarse crepitus, which may be felt by a hand on the joint or occasionally can even be heard. Symptoms of OA include pain related to use of the joint, either while actually using the joint or immediately afterwards and is generally relieved by rest. The pain of OA has an insidious onset and can be variable from day to day. It is variously described as a deep dull ache similar to toothache or as a sharp and severe pain. In more severe and progressive forms of OA, pain becomes more persistent and is present even at rest and at night. Stiffness after inactivity, such as sitting or lying in bed, is another common symptom. This stiffness is short-lasting and will usually have resolved in around 15–30 min. This is sometimes known as 'gelling' of the joints.

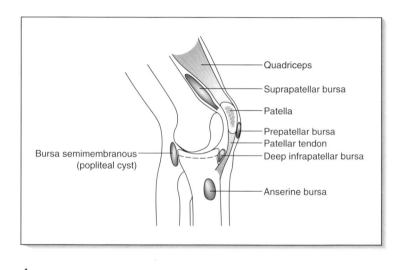

▲

Fig. 1.3 Anserine bursa. Reproduced from Hosie & Field 2002 with permission.

1.22 What causes the pain of OA?

Joint cartilage itself does not contain any pain receptors, but other joint tissues have good sensory innervation. The exact cause of the pain felt in OA is not fully understood but it is thought to be caused by the pathological changes taking place in a number of different structures within and around the joint (*see Box 1.4*).

If there is a sudden acute worsening of pain in an OA joint it is important to consider other causes, such as crystal arthritis (including

---

BOX 1.4 Main pathological changes in and around the OA joint

- Increased pressure within the joint capsule
- Increased pressure within the surrounding bone
- Inflammation of the synovial lining
- Inflammation within the peri-articular structures, such as enthesopathies and bursae
- Peri-osteal changes
- Alteration in the function of the surrounding musculature
- Abnormal pressure on the joint capsule and ligaments

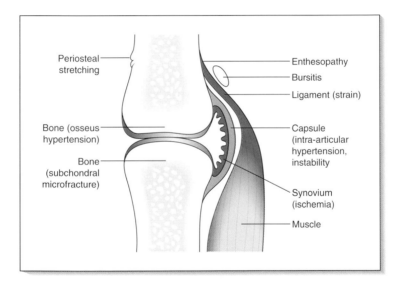

▲

Fig. 1.4 Causes of pain around an OA joint. From Acta Orthopaedica Scandinavica 1994, 65: 375–86 with permission.

gout), septic arthritis or the development of an inflammatory arthritis (*see Fig. 1.4*).

1.23 What causes the stiffness of OA?

The exact cause of the stiffness of OA is not entirely understood, but again it probably reflects the pathological changes within the joint. Possible causes are thickening of the capsule, alteration in the peri-articular structures, accumulation of fluid or patches of synovitis.

1.24 What is crepitus?

In a normal joint, the cartilage-covered ends of bone glide over each other giving a smooth movement. In a joint affected by OA, the joint surfaces become irregular due to breakdown of cartilage and to the growth of osteophytes and chondrocytes at joint margins. When the joint is moved, these irregularities can be felt by a hand over the joint, generally through the full range of movement. In severe OA, crepitus may also be heard as well as felt on movement of the joint. The presence of crepitus is one of a number of diagnostic features included for a diagnosis of OA by the American College of Rheumatology; however, it is not in itself specific to OA and can occur from other causes of joint damage (*see Q. 2.3*).

1.25 What are osteophytes and where are they commonly found?

When a joint sustains damage, one of the repair mechanisms is to form chondrocytes and osteophytes in the areas of fibrocartilage at the margins of the joint. This growth is thought to represent an attempt by the joint to enlarge the area available for articulation and possibly also to assist joint stability. The end result of this growth of osteophytes is to produce visible enlargement of the joint, often leading to the clinical picture of 'squaring of the joints' (*Fig. 1.5*). Heberden's nodes at the distal interphalangeal joints are good examples of the clinical results of the growth of osteophytes at the edges of the joints (*see Fig. 1.6*).

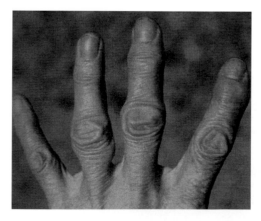

◀ **Fig. 1.5** 'Squaring' of the joint. Reproduced from Hosie & Field 2002 with permission.

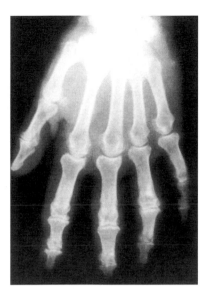

◀ **Fig. 1.6** Heberden's and Bouchard's nodes on X-ray. From University of Bath Diploma in Primary Care Rheumatology 1995 with permission.

1.26 **What are the pathological changes causing impairment of function in a joint affected by OA?**

A number of different pathological changes take place within an OA joint and each can contribute to impairment of function. These include the bony changes of osteophyte growth and the thickening of the joint capsule, both of which may prevent a full range of movement. Effusion within the joint and soft tissue swelling around the joint may contribute to functional impairment. Patients with OA sometimes report a feeling that the joint is giving way; this may be due to impaired function and weakness in the surrounding musculature.

1.27 **What causes swelling in a joint affected by OA and how can you differentiate this from the swelling caused by inflammation or infection?**

The swelling in an OA joint reflects the pathological changes taking place within it. The main cause of the swelling seen in OA is due to the presence of osteophytes at the joint margins. Other causes are thickening of the capsule, peri-articular swelling (perhaps due to bursitis) and occasionally a small cool effusion. The presence of osteophytes gives a firm bony swelling quite different in feel to the soft 'boggy' feeling of synovitis present in inflammatory arthritis. An OA joint is cool and of normal colour and any tenderness is usually confined to the joint line or to peri-articular structures. A joint affected by infection will be red and shiny, will feel hot to touch and will be very tender to touch and to move. A joint affected by inflammation may feel warm, not hot, will show the changes of synovitis and will be tender to palpate or to move.

1.28 What causes the varus angulation sometimes seen in severe OA of the knee?

In chronic severe OA where there is significant destruction of cartilage and underlying bone, obvious joint deformity can occur. When this happens in the medial compartment of the knee it leads to outward bowing of the leg and a typical varus deformity. In inflammatory arthritis, particularly rheumatoid arthritis, the deformity is typically valgus where the leg shows inward bowing.

1.29 What is the prognosis in a patient with OA?

Osteoarthritis generally has an insidious onset and a slow progression. Symptoms may vary, with spells of increased pain and difficulty followed by improvement in function as the joint re-stabilizes. There may be flares of symptoms often related to unaccustomed mechanical stress. Many patients with OA suffer relatively mild symptoms and cope well with their reduced functional capacity, perhaps by making small adaptive changes to their environment. Around 40–50% of those with OA, however, suffer more significant problems with daily pain and disability and require a variety of interventions to deal with their problems. Around 10% of all OA patients become increasingly incapacitated by their condition and suffer severe pain and loss of function and eventually develop end-stage disease. Patients who have OA affecting several joints and who are obese are more likely to develop progressively severe disease.

1.30 At what age should a diagnosis of OA be considered?

There is no specific cut-off age for consideration of OA. In general, OA is uncommon below the age of 50 unless there are specific aggravating features in the history such as previous joint injury or childhood joint problems. The American College Criteria for the classification and reporting of OA of the knee include age over 50 as one of nine parameters, of which five require to be present to satisfy a diagnosis of OA. The other problem is that, in a condition such as OA with a slow insidious onset, it is difficult to identify an exact time for the start of the disease, and patients in younger age groups who present with mild joint problems but without diagnostic criteria may well progress to frank OA over time.

1.31 How many patients develop OA after a menisectomy? Which knee does it affect?

Removal of a meniscus increases the risk of developing OA, presumably by altering the pressure and the tissues within the joint. After a menisectomy, around 50% of patients after 19 years have been found to have OA. OA can occur after both medial and lateral menisectomy, but has been found to be more common with the lateral side. It was also noted that OA in the non-operated knee showed a higher incidence of OA compared to controls, presumably because of slightly altered biomechanics (*see also Ch. 11*).

PQ PATIENT QUESTIONS

1.32 I have OA of my hands and knees. Will my children develop OA?

There is a genetic component to OA of the hands and knees but this does not necessarily mean that your children will develop the condition. They may be able to reduce their risk of developing knee OA by avoiding becoming overweight and keeping active.

1.33 My daughter is double-jointed. Is she more likely to develop OA?

Being double-jointed (also called hypermobile) can cause the joints to extend further than normal and put extra stresses and strains onto them. It is thought that this may make a double-jointed person more likely to develop OA, but there is as yet no definite proof of this. Your daughter should try to protect her joints by warming up before exercise and avoiding overstretching her joints. It is also important to warm down as this will reduce the after-exercise stiffness.

1.34 I am a 45-year-old woman and have recently developed little lumps over the joints at the ends of my fingers. My friend said that this meant that I have OA. I have no problems with my joints at present, but do these lumps mean that I will definitely get OA and can I do anything to stop it?

The lumps you are referring to are called Heberden's nodes. Usually your hands retain very good function, even if they have little lumps on them. The appearance of Heberden's nodes means that you have a genetic tendency to develop OA, particularly of the knee. This does not mean that you will necessarily be badly affected by OA and you can reduce your risk by keeping active and by avoiding becoming overweight. You should also try to protect your knees by avoiding jobs involving kneeling and heavy lifting.

PQ PATIENT QUESTIONS

1.35   I have suffered from pain in my knees for some years and have recently noticed that my knees have become larger and have hard swellings on them. What causes this change of shape?

The changes you describe are due to OA of the knee. In this condition, the bone at the edges of the joints grows outwards and this leads to the appearance of the joint enlarging. The hard swellings that you feel around your knees are also due to these bony enlargements. The swellings themselves, although sometimes unsightly, will do no harm.

1.36   My knees cause me pain when I go up and down stairs, especially going down, and my friend says I must have arthritis. I can walk for miles on the flat with no problems. Do I have arthritis, and is pain going up and down stairs usually the first sign?

There are different areas within the knee joint, and arthritis of each area often has slightly different symptoms. Pain in your knees on going up and down stairs is usually due to arthritis of the joint behind the knee cap or patella. It is important to keep active as you obviously already do and continue your walking as much as possible. If stairs become an increasing problem for you, try to reduce the number of times you have to go up and down and use banisters and railings to help.

Diagnosis of osteoarthritis

2

PQ PATIENT QUESTIONS	
2.21	I attended my GP with pain in my knee. She examined my knee and asked me lots of questions and then told me I had early osteoarthritis in my knee. I asked if I could have an X-ray of my knee but she said it would not be helpful. How can she tell if I do have OA and not some other disease?
2.22	When my friend developed RA she had a lot of blood tests and was put on tablets to stop the disease getting worse. I have been told that I have OA but I have not had any blood tests and have just been given paracetamol. Should I have blood tests and other tablets also?
2.23	My knees make funny grinding noises when I go up or down stairs and I am concerned that I am causing damage to my joints. What causes this noise and does it mean that my arthritis is getting worse?

2.1 What are the criteria for diagnosis of OA?

Diagnostic criteria for OA have been notoriously difficult to define as they may vary according to the affected joint. The American College of Rheumatology definitions of OA of the hip and knee are listed in Box 2.1.

2.2 What are the signs and symptoms of OA in a joint?

Pain in the joint, usually related to use of the joint, is generally the first symptom that brings the patient to the doctor. Pain may be accompanied by stiffness and difficulty in function.
The main signs of OA in a joint are listed in Box 2.2.

2.3 What is crepitus?

When a joint with OA is put through a range of movement with a hand placed over the joint, it is possible to feel a roughness in the movement that

---

BOX 2.1 American College of Rheumatology definitions of OA of the hip and knee (Hochberg et al 1995)

OA of the hip
Hip pain with at least two of the following:

- ESR <20 mm/h
- Radiographic femoral or acetabular osteophytes
- Radiographic joint space narrowing.

OA of the knee
Knee pain and radiographic osteophytes and at least one of the following:

- Age >50 years
- Morning stiffness <30 min in duration
- Crepitus on motion.

BOX 2.2 Signs of OA in a joint

- Decreased range of movement of the joint
- Joint line tenderness
- Bony swelling around the joint due to osteophytes
- Crepitus on movement of the joint
- Occasional deformity of the joint
- Occasional small cool effusion

is unlike the normal smooth movement of a joint. This is what is called crepitus. In severely affected joints, crepitus can be heard as well as felt. Patients sometimes become aware of crepitus, for example in the knee joint, before they develop any real symptoms of pain or disability. Crepitus is thought to be caused by the roughness of the joint surfaces and by osteophytes interfering with the normal smooth joint function.

2.4 Can crepitus occur in normal joints?

Crepitus may occur in joints that do not have OA but which have not been used for some time, perhaps after immobilization due to trauma. It may also occur in joints that to all intents and purposes are normal, with normal X-rays and no abnormal physical signs; this may be related to a minor injury which eventually heals. Some young people may have patellofemoral crepitus on flexion, particularly when weight-bearing, associated with anterior knee pain. This is possibly more common in patients who are hypermobile and may relate to overuse.

2.5 How does the stiffness of OA differ from that of RA?

The stiffness of an OA joint is often described as 'gelling'. This gelling wears off after a few minutes of movement of the joint and is worse after a period of inactivity, such as first thing in the morning or after sitting for some time. The exact cause of the stiffness of OA is not known but possibly relates to some capsular thickening. The stiffness of OA tends to be short-lived and generally lasts for no more than 30 min. Occasionally, patients with severe OA may have stiffness lasting for longer than 30 min; this is thought to be due to a degree of synovitis within the joint.

The stiffness experienced by patients with RA (rheumatoid arthritis) is present on waking in the morning and tends to be much longer, lasting from 1 to 3 h.

2.6 What is the nature of the pain of OA?

The pain of OA tends to be related to movement of the joint and to weight-bearing in affected joints of the lower limb; it is generally relieved by rest. The pain usually has an insidious onset and in the earlier stages of the condition may come and go with long spells in which the patient has very few symptoms followed by spells of increased pain, often related to increased or unaccustomed activity. In later stages of the condition, pain may be present at rest and often in bed at night. The pain of OA is sometimes described as an aching pain and sometimes as an intermittent stabbing pain.

2.7   Is there a pattern of joint involvement in OA and how does this differ from RA?

Joints most commonly affected by OA are the knee, the hip, the distal interphalangeal joints, the carpometacarpal joint of the thumb and the first metatarsophalangeal joint. In RA, the joints most commonly affected are the carpometacarpal, wrist, proximal interphalangeal and metatarsophalangeal joints. The pattern in RA is usually symmetrical, whereas this is not so common in OA where single joints may be affected. RA also occurs quite commonly in knee and shoulder and OA in the sternoclavicular and acromioclavicular joints (*see Fig. 2.1*).

2.8   Some patients with OA of the knee describe a feeling that the knee is going to give way. What is the cause of this feeling?

Many patients with early OA have this feeling of insecurity. This is most likely due to muscle weakness which may be present even in very early disease. This weakness can be treated by specific exercises such as quadriceps exercises. In late disease when there is gross bony abnormality and laxity of the ligaments with stretching of the joint capsule as well as muscle wasting, the knee may well give way for obvious physical reasons.

2.9   What is the differential diagnosis of OA in the knee joint?

The differential diagnosis of knee pain is given in Box 2.3.

2.10   Are there any 'red flags' for knee pain?

Yes there are three particular knee problems that must be excluded in someone presenting with knee pain:

■ Septic arthritis
■ Bony fracture around the joint
■ Major ligamentous injury or internal derangement.

Both fracture and major ligament or meniscal injury will normally be accompanied by a history of trauma and most of these will be referred immediately to hospital.

Septic arthritis usually presents with a hot, swollen and very painful joint which may look shiny and is exquisitely tender to touch or move. The patient usually has systemic symptoms such as fever. Septic arthritis is an extremely serious condition which needs rapid and adequate treatment otherwise it may result in total destruction of the joint and may even be fatal. If septic arthritis is suspected, the

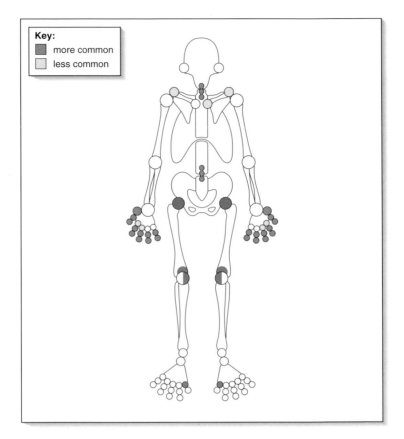

Fig. 2.1 Pattern of joint involvement in OA. From Shipley et al 2002 Rheumatology and bone disease. Based on Kumar P, Clark M (eds) 2002 Clinical medicine, 5th edn. (Saunders).

patient should immediately be referred to hospital. The joint should be aspirated and synovial fluid obtained if possible before starting antibiotic therapy. Initial Gram staining may help to decide on the most appropriate antibiotic, although this may need to be changed depending on the result of the culture. Antibiotic therapy is usually continued for around 4–6 weeks.

Gout can also present with a red, hot, shiny joint that is tender to touch and very painful to move, but in this condition the patient does not usually have constitutional signs of sepsis such as fever. Both septic arthritis and gout generally present as a monoarthritis.

BOX 2.3 Differential diagnosis of knee pain

- Osteoarthritis
- Rheumatoid arthritis (RA)
- Gout
- Pseudogout
- Inflammatory arthritis, including reactive, psoriatic, etc.
- Mechanical disruption within the joint (e.g. meniscal problem)
- Referred pain from hip or knee
- Bursitis, including anserine and prepatellar bursitis
- Sepsis

BOX 2.4 Risk factors for septic arthritis

- Recent intra-articular injection, although sepsis following injection is a very rare occurrence
- Major concomitant illness such as diabetes, RA, malignancy
- Patients with infections such as HIV, gonococcal and systemic infection
- Immunocompromised patients (this includes patients on DMARDs—disease-modifying anti-rheumatic drugs—or biologicals)
- Previous joint replacement with a prosthesis
- Drug addiction

2.11 Are there any specific risk factors for septic arthritis?

There are a number of risk factors which may lead to the suspicion of septic arthritis (*see Box 2.4*). Corticosteroid therapy may mask the signs and symptoms of septic arthritis.

2.12 Can OA and RA occur together?

Yes. RA and OA can occur in the same patient.
   Many older patients have signs and symptoms of OA in their joints, particularly the knee joint. If the patient presents with increasing pain and stiffness in the joint this may be attributed to an exacerbation of OA and treated accordingly, and it is often only when the symptoms worsen and synovitis appears in the index joint and possibly other joints that a diagnosis of RA is suspected. Many patients with long-standing RA develop OA in their hips and knees and may progress to joint replacement.

2.13 How can you distinguish gout from OA?

In OA, the joint may look swollen due to bony osteophytes and capsular thickening and may show joint line tenderness but is not usually red and tender. In acute gout, joint pain is very severe and the joint usually looks red and shiny and is very tender to touch and is generally easy to distinguish from OA. In chronic gout, however, diagnosis may be less clearcut. Chronic gout often affects the proximal interphalangeal joints and distal joint nodes and may occur in patients who have pre-existing OA with Heberden's nodes. Risk factors to consider in chronic gout include introduction of thiazide diuretics for hypertension and recent dietary changes. The patient may already be taking allopurinol to control gout, but the dose may be insufficient to reduce the uric acid level to one which prevents attacks. Whereas acute gout usually affects the first metatarsophalangeal joint, or sometimes knee and ankle, chronic gout is often seen in the hands. Investigations for gout include a serum uric acid level and polarizing microscopy for uric acid crystals in synovial fluid. Note that the uric acid level may be lower during an acute attack and may need to be repeated at a later date to get a true reading. If the patient gets recurrent attacks of acute gout, allopurinol therapy should reduce the uric acid level and prevent recurrence, although the dose may need to be adjusted to prevent attacks of chronic gout. When initiating allopurinol therapy it is important to use concomitant anti-inflammatory or colchicine therapy for the first few weeks of treatment to prevent further attacks of acute gout.

2.14 What investigations should be done on a patient to confirm a diagnosis of OA?

There are no diagnostic tests specific for OA. X-rays can confirm the presence of changes of OA within the joints; however, there is a poor correlation between clinical symptoms and X-ray changes, thus X-rays should not be used as a routine diagnostic tool. X-rays may be useful where there are diagnostic difficulties and where assessment of structural change is important (e.g. when considering joint replacement surgery).

Blood and urine tests are not useful in the diagnosis of OA but may have a place in the differential diagnosis of joint pain and in the exclusion of other conditions. Blood tests may also be used to confirm or exclude the presence of any metabolic condition that could lead to the presence of chondrocalcinosis and to the development of OA in a younger adult. Such metabolic conditions include Wilson's disease, haemochromatosis, hypothyroidism and hyperparathyroidism. Some tests that may be useful in excluding other conditions are listed in Box 2.5.

BOX 2.5 Investigations that could help confirm or exclude a diagnosis of OA

- Serum uric acid. A raised uric acid level is a marker for gout. It is not diagnostic, however, as uric acid may be raised in other conditions such as renal disease and diuretic use.
- Inflammatory markers such as erythrocyte sedimentation rate (ESR), C-reactive protein (CRP). OA by itself does not produce rises in inflammatory markers. If levels of these markers are raised and signs and symptoms are appropriate, this could suggest inflammatory joint disease. If the clinical picture suggests OA but the inflammatory markers are raised, this could suggest another, unrelated, cause.
- Rheumatoid factor (RF). RF is not specific for rheumatoid arthritis and can occur in normal individuals. Only around 70% of patients with RA have a positive RF. If RF is found in high titres and the clinical picture supports, then the likely diagnosis is RA.
- Synovial fluid analysis. There are no specific changes in synovial fluid relating to OA. There may be a place for aspiration of synovial fluid to exclude crystal arthritis or septic arthritis.

2.15   Can fibromyalgia be confused with OA?

Patients with fibromyalgia often present complaining of pain all over and associated stiffness, and describe more generalized pain than that specifically relating to joints. Patients with fibromyalgia are usually aged under 50 and often suffer from other conditions such as headache, tiredness, irritable bowel and poor sleep pattern. Examination may show tender points (*see Fig. 2.2*). Patients with generalized OA are usually aged over 50 with use-related pain and signs of OA in the joints. Older patients with OA who complain of generalized pain may be suffering from depression.

2.16   What is pseudogout and how can it be distinguished from OA?

Pseudogout is caused by pyrophosphate crystals being released from articular cartilage. This causes acute pain and stiffness, usually in a single joint. It is most commonly seen in the wrist and knee joints and may be triggered by an insult to the body such as surgery, trauma or illness. It may occur in joints already affected by OA. It usually occurs in patients over 70 years old. There may be a genetic predisposition to develop this condition, or it may be associated with endocrine and metabolic conditions such as haemochromatosis, hypothyroidism and hypercalcaemia. X-rays may show chondrocalcinosis (linear calcification in articular cartilage) together with

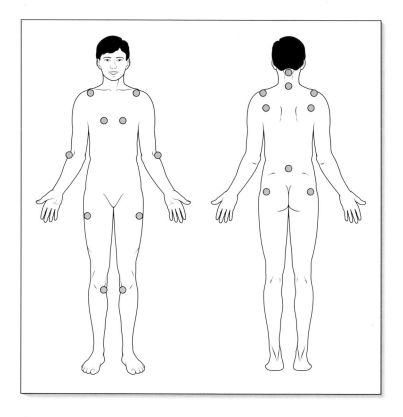

▲

Fig. 2.2 Sites of tenderness in patients with fibromyalgia. From Hosie & Field 2002 with permission.

underlying OA. The joints often have effusions which should be aspirated, and the synovial fluid examined with a polarizing microscope for crystals and sent for culture to exclude sepsis.

2.17 **Can there be physical signs of OA in a joint that is asymptomatic?**

Some patients show both physical and radiological signs of OA without experiencing very much in the way of symptoms. In the longer term, however, most of these patients will develop some pain and/or stiffness. Patients vary enormously in their acceptance of mild disability and pain and many older patients feel that some joint pain is inevitable with increasing age and accept this as an almost normal state.

2.18 Is pain always the first sign of OA?

Pain is usually the first symptom that brings the patient to the doctor. If an X-ray is performed at this time there may well be considerable radiological signs of OA within the joint even at this early stage (*see Q2.2*).

2.19 When an X-ray report states 'moderate degenerative changes present' what does this mean in radiological terms?

'Moderate degenerative changes' usually means that there are osteophytes present together with moderate reduction of the joint space. 'Minimal degenerative changes' means that there is a definite osteophyte but the joint space is not reduced. 'Severe degenerative changes' means the presence of osteophytes and severe reduction of joint space, together with sclerosis of the subchondral bone. Cysts in the subchondral bone may occur in moderate to severe OA.

2.20 Can a primary care physician make a confident diagnosis of OA?

Yes. If a primary care physician takes a good history and makes a careful examination of the joints and is aware of common patterns of joint problems and of other potential diagnoses that may need to be excluded, then there is no reason why he or she should not be able to make a diagnosis of OA. As OA is such a common problem, primary care physicians develop considerable expertise in examining joints affected by OA and are well placed to make a confident diagnosis and to manage the condition within primary care, with appropriate referral to other agencies as required.

PQ PATIENT QUESTIONS

2.21 I attended my GP with pain in my knee. She examined my knee and asked me lots of questions and then told me I had early osteoarthritis in my knee. I asked if I could have an X-ray of my knee but she said it would not be helpful. How can she tell if I do have OA and not some other disease?

By asking you questions and examining your knee, your GP would be able to tell a lot about your knee problem. Not only would she be able to diagnose probable osteoarthritis, she would also be able to tell that you did not have other potentially serious conditions in your knee. To try to limit harmful radiation from X-rays, doctors try only to X-ray if necessary and if the result is likely to alter the management of your condition.

2.22   When my friend developed RA she had a lot of blood tests and was put on tablets to stop the disease getting worse. I have been told that I have OA but I have not had any blood tests and have just been given paracetamol. Should I have blood tests and other tablets also?

When your friend developed RA she would have had a variety of blood tests to confirm the diagnosis and to monitor the severity of the inflammation in her joints. When a patient develops RA, he or she is treated with a slow-acting or disease-modifying drug to try to limit the inflammation within the joints and to reduce the long-term damage to the joints. As yet there are no blood tests to confirm the diagnosis of OA or to monitor any change in the condition and we do not have any drugs that can change the long-term outlook. There is some evidence that glucosamine (which you can buy from chemists and health food shops) may prevent some long-term damage due to OA in some individuals but the evidence is not yet clear-cut.

2.23   My knees make funny grinding noises when I go up or down stairs and I am concerned that I am causing damage to my joints. What causes this noise and does it mean that my arthritis is getting worse?

The noise you hear from your knees is called crepitus. This is due to the joint surfaces within your joint becoming roughened due to your OA. It is important to keep moving and to use your joints; sensible exercise will not cause further damage to your knee joints. If you are unsure about the sort of exercise you should be taking ask your doctor for advice.

Joint examination

3

GENERAL JOINT EXAMINATION

3.1 What do OA joints feel like?

Normal joints are relatively hard and we know the shape of our own, as we often feel them and look at them subconsciously. Osteoarthritic joints feel harder, and tend to be nearer the surface, as an OA joint is larger than the normal one. If large joints are affected by OA, it is rarely possible to feel the osteophytes that are seen on X-ray, so the joint feels relatively smooth and the normal bony ridges are more pronounced. This is not true for hand joints, as Heberden's and Bouchard's nodes are osteophytes and can be easily felt and seen. Most OA joints become squarer; for example, the knee joint changes from having a triangular profile to having a large square profile (*see Fig. 1.5*). Similarly, the carpometacarpal joint of the thumb looks square when affected by OA. If the right and left sides of the body are both affected by OA, the dominant side is often more severely affected.

3.2 How does the feel of an OA joint compare to the feel of an RA joint?

A joint affected by rheumatoid arthritis (RA) feels softer and looks more swollen than a normal or an OA joint. Importantly, even normal examination pressure may be painful; certainly squeezing the joint is! Often the normal contours and prominences are difficult to identify. This is because the characteristic pathology of RA—the proliferating synovium—has distended the joint capsule, so the feel is of bogginess rather than hardness. There will be a major difference in joint movement and function between OA and RA. Movement of an OA joint will be slower than a normal joint and often will produce crepitus, which can be felt and even heard. RA movement will be even slower and often painful. Importantly, joint function is severely compromised; for example, patients with RA affecting their hands will drop cups on a regular basis every day, whereas patients with OA hands will drop the occasional cup during the week. Patients with OA knees will find it difficult to bend or kneel but the RA patient will not kneel because it is far too painful and almost impossible to get back up, as the joint movement is so slow and painful.

3.3 How do joints in a patient with fibromyalgia differ from RA and OA joints?

The feel of joints in fibromyalgia patients is quite different from that in OA or RA joints. They feel normal, and when they are moved passively they move normally. The patient may complain of early morning stiffness and swelling of the hand joints. This swelling is subjective, as the joints, when examined, do not feel swollen and move freely when moved through the range of motion by the examiner. This is the key, as active movements by the patient may be slower and they may complain of pain when gripping things tightly or when the examiner squeezes the joint. This is because patients with fibromyalgia have pain augmentation for normal sensations of touch and pressure.

3.4 Why should we examine our patients' joints?

Even when we are sure from a history that we are dealing with OA in a joint, it is important to examine the joints both at the initial visit and at review visits for various reasons (*see Box 3.1*).

HIP EXAMINATION

3.5 Where is the pain of OA in the hip most commonly felt?

Classically the pain of OA hip is felt in the groin area and most patients presenting with OA of the hip will complain of pain in this area, although they may also complain of pain in the lateral aspect of the hip and thigh and around the buttock. The pain may also be felt in the front of the thigh. Sometimes hip pain can be referred to the knee, although this is less common.

3.6 What (other) pain sites can be felt around hip joints?

In a patient with pain due to OA of the hip, the pain is classically felt in the groin, although it can also be felt in surrounding areas (*see Q. 3.5*) and can occasionally be referred to the knee. If a patient complaining of knee pain has a completely normal knee on examination, remember to check hip movements. Pain around the hip can also arise from inflammation of some of the bursae in this area, in particular the trochanteric, subtrochanteric, adductor and ischial bursae (*see Fig. 3.1*). If a patient presents with bursitis, particularly trochanteric bursitis, remember to check hip movements, as

---

BOX 3.1 Why it is important to examine the joints at all visits

- ■ To establish a diagnosis
- ■ To exclude 'red flags'
- ■ To exclude referred pain
- ■ To assess progression
- ■ To establish whether any other condition has arisen in a joint previously diagnosed with OA
- ■ To provide confidence and reassurance to our patients

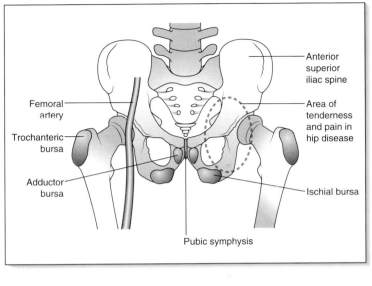

Femoral
artery

Trochanteric
bursa

Adductor
bursa

Anterior
superior
iliac spine

Area of
tenderness
and pain in
hip disease

Ischial bursa

Pubic symphysis

Fig. 3.1 Diagram to show the bursae round the hip. From Hosie & Field 2002 with permission.

trochanteric bursitis is often associated with OA of the hip. It is thought that bursitis occurs as a result of abnormal pressure exerted because of OA within the joint.

3.7 How are hip movements examined?

Hip movements are best examined with the patient lying supine on the couch, although a simpler method to check passive hip rotation can be used with the patient sitting. The two most sensitive movements to test are rotation and hip flexion.

To examine hip flexion with the patient supine, ask the patient to flex the knee and then push the thigh up over the abdomen. A normal value for hip flexion is 135°. To examine hip rotation with the patient supine, flex both hip and knee to 90° and, using the lower leg as a pointer, move the foot and ankle medially and laterally (*see Fig. 3.2*). Normal values for full hip rotation are 35° for internal rotation and 45° for external rotation. Moving the foot laterally in this position tests internal rotation of the hip joint; moving it medially tests external rotation.

To examine the patient in the seated position, ask the patient to sit on the couch or high chair with legs hanging and slightly parted. An ordinary

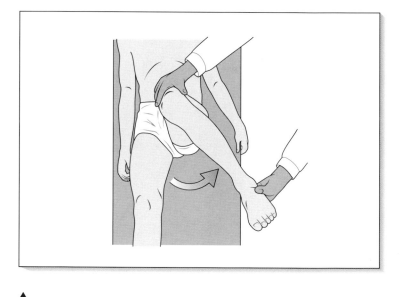

▲

Fig. 3.2 Testing hip rotation with the patient in the supine position. From Hosie & Field 2002 with permission.

chair is not appropriate, as the legs cannot hang and measurements may be inaccurate. Again using the lower leg as a pointer, keeping the hip and knee stationary, move the foot outwards and inwards. Moving the foot outwards tests internal rotation of the hip; moving it inwards tests external rotation.

These movements can be measured, if required, using a plurimeter, but for most practical purposes the sense of limitation of movement is all that is required. Examining the patient seated is possibly less sensitive than examining the patient supine, but it may be more convenient, easier for the patient and more appropriate in a busy practice. If movements are being measured with a plurimeter, the seated method is preferable, as it is easier to find neutral (i.e. with the lower leg hanging). When measuring internal and external rotation with the patient seated, it is important to make sure that the hips are stabilized; otherwise, you may get a false reading as the patient moves the whole body and tilts the pelvis at the limit of internal rotation. It is therefore advisable to ask the patient to place hands on hips so that any tilting can be seen by the examiner.

If the patient has a knee problem, such as OA, and is unable to flex the knee, this may give an incorrect value of hip flexion.

3.8   Which movements of the hip are affected by OA?

Internal rotation is the earliest and most sensitive sign of hip OA. Progressive loss of hip internal rotation indicates worsening of OA, although occasionally some patients can show practically no internal rotation on examination and have only moderate and slowly progressive symptoms. Flexion is also reduced in hip OA.

3.9   What is the Thomas test?

Disease of the hip often leads to a fixed flexion deformity and manifests itself by the patient limping. To examine for this, use the Thomas test. Ask the patient to lie supine and fully flex the normal hip. If there is a fixed flexion deformity, the thigh will be raised from the couch and the knee will flex (*see Fig. 3.3*).

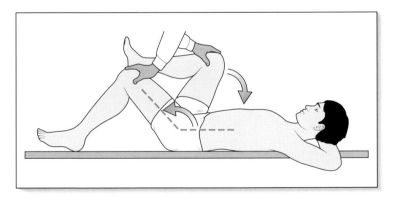

▲

Fig. 3.3 The Thomas test. From University of Bath Diploma in Primary Care Rheumatology 1995 with permission.

3.10   What is the Trendelenburg test?

The Trendelenburg test tests the strength of the abductor muscles of the hip. With a normal hip, when the patient puts the weight onto one hip and lifts the other leg off the ground, the pelvis tilts and rises on the non-weight-bearing side. In OA of the hip, the hip abductors may become weak,

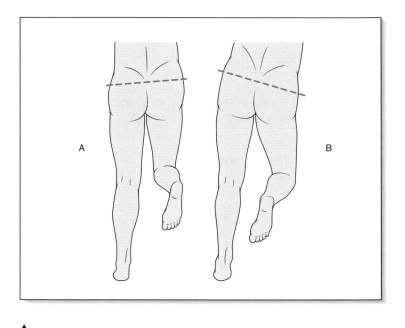

▲

Fig. 3.4 The Trendelenburg test, distinguishing pelvic tilt of a normal hip (a) and that of an OA hip (b). From University of Bath Diploma in Primary Care Rheumatology 1995 with permission.

due to pain, and this causes a drop in the pelvis on the unaffected side when the patient puts weight on the affected side (*see Fig. 3.4*).

3.11 What can be learnt from watching a patient walk?

In hip disease, patients often present complaining of pain and a limp. Fixed flexion deformity (*see Q. 3.9*) gives an antalgic gait. Because of pain, the patient is uncomfortable when putting weight on the affected hip and 'hurries off it'. When pain causes weakness of the hip abductors, the patient is unable to tilt the pelvis when putting weight on the affected side and this gives a Trendelenburg gait (*see Q. 3.10*). Most abnormal gaits that are due to hip disease will present as a mixture of antalgic and Trendelenburg gaits. If both hips are affected, this can produce a rolling gait, which again is a mixture of both antalgic and Trendelenburg gaits.

EXAMINATION OF THE KNEE

3.12 What are the steps in examination of the knee?

First, look at the knee. Look for any abnormalities of shape or colour. If the patient has knee OA, you may notice 'squaring' of the joint due to bony osteophytes. If there is an obvious large effusion or the joint is red, remember to exclude 'red flags' such as infection, trauma and inflammatory joint disease. If there is OA in the knee, you may see wasting of the quadriceps muscle; this can be present even in early knee OA. Remember to compare the two knees.

Now feel the joint for bony structures and for joint line tenderness. You should also feel around the joint as there may be soft tissue lesions, such as bursitis, associated with OA. The anserine bursa, which lies medially below the knee, often develops inflammation associated with OA. Effusions may also be present and can be tested (*see Q. 3.18*). You should then move the joint throughout its range of movement and feel for crepitus at the same time. If you suspect a knee stability problem you can test for this (*see Q. 3.22*).

3.13 What does a knee joint with OA look and feel like?

A knee with OA tends to look squarer and larger than a normal joint. It is hard on palpation, and quadriceps muscle wasting may be present. If there is severe long-standing knee OA, a varus deformity may be present, or a fixed flexion deformity where the patient is unable to straighten the knee.

3.14 Do patients with knee OA develop meniscal problems?

Yes, and they do so from much less severe activity in comparison to younger people, such as a twisting injury when playing with the grandchildren. Meniscal problems should be considered as a cause of pain and swelling in the patient who has tripped or stumbled when walking over uneven ground; and don't forget modern shopping areas often have sections of cobbles. Patients present, as expected, with knee swelling and often some pain. The swelling is due to an effusion (*see Q. 3.18*), which is usually straw-coloured on aspiration and often recurs. It should not have blood in it; a bloody effusion signifies more severe damage.

3.15 Which meniscus is commonly injured in OA?

In sports people, the medial meniscus is commonly involved, whereas in patients with OA it is more likely to be the lateral meniscus. It is said that

---

BOX 3.2 Signs and symptoms of meniscal problems
- Locking
- Limited extension
- Joint line tenderness, which may be present at different degrees of flexion
- Grating rather than crepitus
- Effusion, which may be acute or recurrent
- Quadriceps wasting, which is often more severe than expected

---

chronic stress injuries more commonly affect the lateral meniscus. Mucoid degeneration may take place in the lateral meniscus and a meniscal cyst can develop. This cyst will be seen on full extension and should not be confused with a ganglion, a bursa or even an effusion. Knees with meniscal problems grate, and crepitus may not be felt. It is important to check quadriceps, as wasting is often worse than would be expected from the severity of the OA.

3.16   What are the signs and symptoms of meniscal problems?

See Box 3.2.

3.17   If you suspect a meniscal problem on the basis of signs and symptoms, what should your management be?

You should refer the patient for further investigation, such as MRI (magnetic resonance imaging) or arthroscopy, to assess any internal joint damage.

3.18   How are effusions detected in knee joints?

There are two common ways to examine for effusions (*see Box 3.3*).

3.19   What is anterior knee pain?

Anterior knee pain in patients aged over 45 is most usually due to patellofemoral OA. In young patients, especially females, anterior knee pain may be due to overactivity in sports and chondromalacia patellae may be seen on arthroscopy. In this age group, anterior knee pain syndrome is best treated by physiotherapy, strapping, appropriate footwear and avoidance of athletic activity. It is often difficult to treat and may persist for several months.

Patellofemoral OA often presents with increasing knee pain on going down stairs and with significant crepitus. The joint may appear almost normal, with less squaring than might be expected from the history, and may show considerable tenderness on the lateral border of the patella.

BOX 3.3 Two methods to examine for effusions

The patellar tap test

This is useful for moderate to large effusions; usually at least 20 mL of fluid would be present when this test is positive.

Method

Using your non-dominant hand, squash the fluid from the suprapatellar pouch to behind the patella, leave your hand over the pouch, using your thumb or a finger of your dominant hand, press sharply over the centre of the patella (as if playing a piano note). This moves the patella onto the femur below (this has been given the name balloting). The patella will oscillate between your finger and femur. This will allow you to gauge the size of the effusion.

The swipe test

This test (also known as the bulge or cross-fluctuation test) is especially useful for detecting small effusions. In fact a good technique will detect excess fluid of around 10 mL.

Method

Use your thumb to stabilize the patella and stroke downwards on the medial compartment. This is to move all fluid into the lateral compartment or lateral gutter. Now with the patella still stabilized, swipe the lateral compartment and look for a bulge of the medial compartment.

3.20 How is anterior knee pain tested?

Ask the patient to lie flat on the examination couch. Push the patella onto the femoral condyle. If there is significant patellofemoral OA, this procedure may produce pain. If you then keep pressing and ask the patient to contract the quadriceps muscle, this will reproduce the patellofemoral pain. This procedure may be excruciatingly painful for the patient so you should proceed cautiously.

3.21 How do we assess a patient who complains of a feeling that their knee is about to give way or indeed has given way causing them to stumble?

Check the range of movement of the joint and compare both sides. Check anterior/posterior stability using the 'draw' test to test the integrity of the cruciate ligaments (*see Q. 3.22*) and check also the integrity of the collateral ligaments (*see Q. 3.24*). Remember that, even in early OA, a feeling of instability is probably due to muscle weakness.

3.22 How is knee stability tested?

To test the integrity of the cruciate ligaments, use the draw test. Ask the patient to lie on the examination couch with the hip flexed at 45° and the knee at 90°. Place your hands posteriorly behind the tibia and pull forwards. This tests the anterior cruciate ligament and is known as the anterior draw test (*see Fig. 3.5*). Too much movement present would suggest

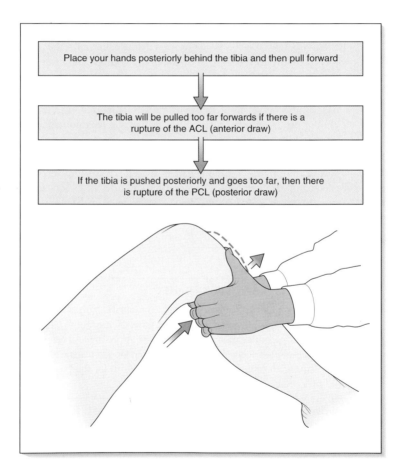

Place your hands posteriorly behind the tibia and then pull forward

The tibia will be pulled too far forwards if there is a rupture of the ACL (anterior draw)

If the tibia is pushed posteriorly and goes too far, then there is rupture of the PCL (posterior draw)

▲

Fig. 3.5 The anterior draw test. From University of Bath Diploma in Primary Care Rheumatology 1995 with permission.

instability and possibly a ruptured anterior cruciate ligament. To test the posterior cruciate ligament, the tibia is pushed posteriorly. Similarly, too much movement here would suggest a ruptured posterior cruciate ligament.

3.23 Are tests for knee stability easily performed by non-specialists?

On the face of it, the tests (*see Q. 3.22*) would appear easy to perform. This is probably true for very unstable knees, but in those with more minor degrees of instability and in those with good musculature these tests are very difficult to perform and to interpret in primary care as few of us see sufficient patients to become really proficient. If you have any doubt about stability based on history and examination, it is best to refer for further investigation.

3.24 How do you test the integrity of the collateral ligaments of the knee?

Ask the patient to lie supine on the examination couch. Flex the knee to about 30° to relax the posterior capsule and the posterior cruciate ligament. To test the lateral collateral ligament, apply pressure to the medial side of the knee joint; reverse the procedure to test the medial collateral ligament. Assess whether there is any looseness or rocking at the joint.

EXAMINATION OF THE FOOT AND ANKLE

3.25 How are the joints of the foot and ankle examined?

Pain in the foot is common, and when examining a foot we should be looking for signs of a variety of conditions (*see Box 3.4*).

Many of these conditions can be suspected from the patient's history. OA can occur in the foot but it is not one of the most common sites. OA in the foot often evolves secondary to past trauma and to biomechanical factors such as inappropriate footwear.

BOX 3.4 Conditions that can cause pain in the foot

- Mechanical and structural conditions, such as pronated or flat foot and supinated or claw foot
- OA
- Soft tissue conditions, such as tendonitis, plantar fasciitis, etc.
- Inflammatory joint disease, such as RA
- Gout
- Diabetes
- Traumatic lesions, such as stress fracture
- Morton's or interdigital neuroma

Look first at the patient's feet with the patient sitting and then standing, to check supination and pronation of the foot. Look also for swelling, discolouration and deformity. It is useful also to look at the patient's feet from behind with the patient standing, to assess supination/pronation.

To examine the ankle joint, which is a hinge joint between the tibia and fibula and the talus, you should hold the lower leg at the back proximal to the malleoli and move the foot with your other hand (*see Fig. 3.6*). This joint permits only flexion and extension (sometimes called plantar flexion and dorsiflexion); full flexion is around 45° degrees and full extension around 20°.

The next joint to examine in the foot is the subtalar or talocalcaneal joint. This joint allows inversion and eversion of the foot and is examined by stabilizing the lower leg with one hand and rocking the calcaneus from side to side. Normal movements here are 30° for inversion and 20° for eversion.

The next joint area to assess is at the midfoot, where there is a composite set of joints which act together to provide rotation, normally about 30° of inversion and 40° of eversion. To test this joint, stabilize the lower leg and hindfoot by holding the calcaneum with one hand and rotating the midfoot with the other hand.

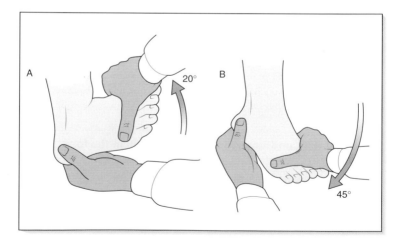

▲

Fig. 3.6 Examination of the ankle joint: (a) dorsiflexion, (b) plantar flexion. From University of Bath Diploma in Primary Care Rheumatology 1995 with permission.

The most common area of the foot to develop OA is the first metatarsophalangeal joint. OA may also develop in the talonavicular and the calcaneocuboid joints but rarely in the ankle or subtalar joints unless secondary to trauma.

3.26 How does examination distinguish between OA and gout of the big toe?

In both gout and OA of the first metatarsophalangeal joint there may be swelling and some redness. In gout, the redness tends to be very significant with the overlying skin shiny and tense. The joint feels hot and is usually extremely tender and the patient is reluctant for the joint to be touched. In OA, if there is redness it is usually milder and often due to the pressure from an ill-fitting shoe. In OA, the joint can be moved through flexion and extension where the range of movement will be found to be reduced and crepitus will often be felt. This may produce some discomfort for the patient but nothing like the pain caused in a joint with gout.

3.27 Is it the bunion or the OA of the first metatarsophalangeal that brings the patient to the doctor?

Bunions are generally caused by underlying OA of the first metatarsophalangeal joint which eventually leads to a rotational deformity of the toe leading to a hallux valgus. Bunions may be aggravated by unsuitable footwear which presses on this area and causes the deformity to enlarge, often getting to the stage where almost any form of footwear is uncomfortable. At this stage surgery is the usual option. OA in this joint does not always lead to the development of bunions, and many patients have primary OA of this joint with little in the way of symptoms. Less commonly, some patients develop hallux rigidus where large osteophytes develop and limit extension of the joint and therefore interfere with walking.

EXAMINATION OF THE UPPER LIMB

3.28 How does examination help differentiate OA of the shoulders from other causes of shoulder pain?

There is no definitive examination for OA of the shoulder as this condition is often accompanied by rotator cuff and subacromial pathology giving a mixed picture of signs. OA of the glenohumeral joint of the shoulder is not very common but does occur in the elderly, particularly elderly women. Signs of OA of the shoulder include anterior joint line tenderness, crepitus, decreased range of movement—particularly abduction and external rotation—and wasting of the surrounding muscles. If shoulder problems do not resolve following appropriate steroid injections for capsulitis or impingement problems, it is worth considering a diagnosis of OA and referring for an X-ray. If there is significant OA of the glenohumeral joint and the patient is symptomatic, then it is worth referring for a surgical opinion and possible arthroplasty.

If there is a large effusion present, this could be due to crystal arthropathy associated with severe OA ('Milwaukee shoulder') or to inflammatory arthritis. 'Milwaukee shoulder' is usually found in elderly women and is associated with the presence of apatite crystals.

3.29 What will be found on examination of the sternoclavicular and acromioclavicular joints with OA?

OA of both these joints is quite common and when present shows the usual signs of bony swelling and crepitus and often tenderness over the joint. The cardinal sign of OA of the acromioclavicular is a positive 'scarf' test. The patient is asked to flex the shoulder and move the arm across the front of the chest to the opposite shoulder as if throwing a scarf around the neck (*see Fig. 3.7*). This movement and that of raising the arm above 90° of abduction stresses the joint and gives rise to pain if there is OA present. OA of the acromioclavicular joint is common in the older age groups, and the signs can be confounded by the existence of associated rotator cuff pathology. In younger patients, OA of this joint may relate to previous injury from rugby or throwing sports, for example, or to overuse as in wheelchair users. OA of the sternoclavicular may present with pain and a warm swelling over the joint. If this occurs the joint should be aspirated to exclude sepsis and crystal joint disease.

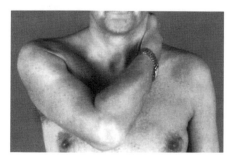

◀ **Fig. 3.7** 'Scarf' test to assess the acromioclavicular joint. Reproduced from Hosie & Field 2002 with permission.

3.30 How do you examine for OA of the elbow?

Elbow OA is not common but may occur following trauma. Signs of OA of the elbow include reduction of both flexion and extension and of pronation and supination. There may also be a fixed flexion deformity. Pain is usually fairly well localized to the elbow but may radiate to the forearm.

3.31 What are the common signs of OA in the hand?

> Patients often present asking about Heberden's nodes and Bouchard's nodes. These nodes are the commonest presenting signs of hand OA. Some patients present with swollen metacarpophalangeal joints, especially the second and third joints (*see also Q. 3.32*).

3.32 How does examination help differentiate the patterns of hand OA?

Examination of patients who have hand OA will differentiate five patterns (*see Box 3.5*).

BOX 3.5 The five patterns of hand OA

Type I: Heberden's and Bouchard's nodes

- Patients may present with painful nodes, usually only when they are developing; the nodes may be inflamed and swollen
- Finger and thumb movements are not affected
- Grip is not affected and function only minimally
- In the very elderly, gout may superimpose on the distal interphalangeal nodes and joints
- Treatment is rarely required; a topical NSAID (non-steroidal anti-inflammatory drug) may help, or rarely a small quantity of triamcinolone can be injected

Type II: Squaring of the first carpometacarpal thumb joint (CMC)

- Thumb pain which is use-related
- CMC joint is square
- Dominant hand is affected first
- Patient's grip and power grip is affected so that the twisting grip is painful
- Often no other joint is affected
- Usually excellent response to steroid injections
- CMC splints may be used for hobbies (e.g. gardening)

BOX 3.5 The five patterns of hand OA (*cont'd*)

Type III: Stiff, thick fingers

■ Wide and thicker fingers

■ Distal interphalangeal, interphalangeal and metacarpophalangeal (MCP) joints may show squaring

■ Thumb joints are usually spared

■ Function and movements, especially apposition of fingers into the palm of the hand, greatly affected by increased tissue in and around the flexor sheaths

■ Usually both hands are affected to a varying degree

■ Holding golf clubs, tools and cups difficult

■ This is not the same as Dupuytren's contracture

■ If seen early enough (e.g. before they have given up golf), then injections into the flexor sheaths may restore function and grip

Type IV(a): Painful swollen knuckles

■ Patients present with painful MCP joints, usually the index and middle fingers

■ There is moderate inflammatory swelling of the involved MCP joints

■ Joints painful to palpation as well as movement

■ Thumb CMC joints often painful but rarely inflamed

■ Grip is severely affected so patient has great difficulty with cups, cutlery and buttons

■ Commonly seen in people over 65 who knit

■ These MCP joints respond well to steroid injections, which may be given intermittently

Type IV(b): Painful swollen knuckles and thumbs

■ A more severe presentation of type IV(a)

■ Most MCP and first CMC joints are painful and swollen

■ Interphalangeal joints also involved, being painful and swollen

■ Both hands are generally equally affected and swollen

■ Gripping and power grip difficult and extremely painful

■ There is NO constitutional upset (in contrast to RA)

■ No sweaty palms (in contrast to RA)

■ May affect both men and women

■ Usually seen in people who work manually

■ There are too many joints to inject

■ Most patients respond well to small doses of sulfasalazine (1 g daily), although a few require 3 g daily; hydroxychloroquine is an alternative (200 mg on 5 days a week)

BOX 3.5 The five patterns of hand OA (*cont'd*)

Type V: Deformed hands with good function

■ Hands show ulnar deviation of joints and ulnar drift

■ All joints are affected

■ Usually have both Heberden's and Bouchard's nodes

■ MCP joints are swollen and the first CMC joints are square

■ Wrist joints may be involved, showing limited, painful movement; sometimes there is even some ankylosis of the wrist joints

■ Can be mistaken for RA but:

—Little loss of function (cf. RA)

—Grip strength retained

—Flares caused by knocks of working

—Flares respond to analgesics or an appropriate steroid injection

—All inflammatory markers are negative

■ X-ray reports may report erosion in unstable distal interphalangeal OA; but these erosions are central, not peripheral as in RA, so view the X-rays or ask for clarification to avoid erroneous diagnosis or treatment

---

Non-pharmacological management 1: General management, educational and environmental issues

4

GENERAL MANAGEMENT AND ASSESSMENT OF OA

4.1 What are the steps in the management of a patient with OA?

The main aims in the management of OA are to

- Reduce pain
- Optimize function
- Provide education and information
- Advise about prevention of further damage.

The first step is to provide information and education about OA and its likely prognosis. The more patients understand about their condition the better they are able to cope with the problems of a potentially painful chronic disease. Some of the points to emphasize at this time are:

- The nature of the condition
- The probable good prognosis
- Lifestyle modifications (*see Box 4.1*) and self-management options
- The fact that there are many treatment options available.

Patients should also be advised about simple analgesia, in particular regular use of paracetamol (*see Ch. 7*). Other simple pain-relief strategies include use of heat and cold and topical rubs and gels, and possibly glucosamine. If pain is more severe, other pharmacological remedies may be appropriate (*see Chs 7–10*).

Physiotherapy treatment may be appropriate for some patients at this stage (*see Q. 5.7*).

4.2 Can OA be prevented?

At present there are no drugs or other treatments that will prevent the development of OA. In patients who have known risk factors, such as a genetic tendency, previous trauma to a joint, or previous childhood problems in a joint, removal of known aggravating factors (e.g. obesity,

---

BOX 4.1 Areas in which advice about lifestyle modification should be given

- Weight loss if overweight
- Suitable exercise, including both aerobic exercise and more specific exercises such as quadriceps strengthening for knee OA (*see Qs 5.2 and 5.6*)
- Suitable footwear (*see Q. 5.11*)
- Pacing activities (*see Q. 4.8*)

unsuitable occupation) may help. In those who have no obvious risk factors, the best advice we can give at present is to keep active, avoid occupations or sports known to aggravate OA and to maintain a normal body weight. There has been a suggestion in the trials on glucosamine that there may be a reduction in joint space loss. However, these studies are not really conclusive of a preventive role for glucosamine and certainly there is no justification for using the drug in this way.

4.3   Is it possible to influence the outcome in patients with already established symptomatic OA?

There are some measures that can help patients who are already suffering pain and loss of function from OA, although they are not always effective in changing the outcome. The first approach should be to provide education and explanation regarding the nature of the condition and try to involve the patient in some decision-making. Advice to lose weight is often ignored by obese patients because of lack of knowledge regarding diet as well as lack of determination. If you can give patients practical advice on diet and arrange follow-up as encouragement this often has a very positive outcome. There are studies showing that a weight loss of 5 kg in overweight women with a body mass index of 25 or over resulted in lack of radiographic progression as well as a reduction of around 50% in pain scores; this background information is worth showing to patients so that they can see that there may be a positive outcome in terms of symptoms. Exercise has been shown to be beneficial for all joints, including those already damaged by OA, and patients should be encouraged to start and maintain an exercise programme designed to improve muscle function around the joint. If possible, this is best started by a physiotherapist, but if this is not practical then the patient can be shown simple exercises such as quadriceps strengthening by a doctor or practice nurse. Both losing weight and exercising are fairly boring and many patients do not manage to keep their original good intentions. For this reason it is very important to give follow-up appointments to try to maintain motivation; even a follow-up phone call has been shown to help.

Many patients will gain some benefit from these lifestyle interventions and may require less analgesic medication. For others, however, despite losing weight and maintaining an exercise programme, there may be little improvement in symptoms. Sometimes, despite all the best efforts of the patient, OA progresses and causes increasing pain and disability.

4.4   Are there any successful strategies for helping overweight patients with lower-limb OA to lose weight?

The first important factor is to try to motivate the patient. Although you can advise that for many patients with OA there will be an improvement in symptoms with weight loss, obviously you cannot promise that this will be the case for any individual but it is certainly worthwhile trying. Having encouraged the patient to try to lose weight it is important to keep providing support in the longer term. Even with highly motivated patients there will be spells where they become discouraged as weight loss slows, so support is vital at this stage. It is also important to provide dietary advice, either from a dietician or from the practice team. Despite much publicity about healthy eating and the fat content of food, many patients have only a scant idea about nutrition and often need fairly basic guidelines to help them plan a weight-loss programme. Weight loss should be accompanied by an increase in exercise if possible; even patients who have significant symptomatic OA can often increase the amount of exercise in their daily activities. Again, support is often needed for an exercise programme and most patients appreciate suggestions as how to build this up over a period of time.

4.5 How should we advise a patient with newly diagnosed knee OA?

First, we should make sure that the patient understands something about the nature of OA, including the fact that OA differs from rheumatoid arthritis (RA), the likely prognosis of OA, the fact that there are a large number of different treatment options and that the patient can do much to help him- or herself by lifestyle changes. The aims of management are to provide information to help the patient cope with the condition, to provide pain control as required, to suggest a programme of exercise to improve movement and to prevent further damage to the knee joints. At this early stage in the condition it is really important to help the patient to develop a positive attitude to the condition and to suggest ways in which the individual can take control of his or her own treatment and become involved in their own decision-making. Many patients appreciate information leaflets that they can take away and read at home. Both the Primary Care Rheumatology Society and the Arthritis Research Campaign (*see Appendix 3*) produce leaflets for patients specifically on knee OA, and it is well worth having some in your consulting room for this common condition.

4.6 What exercise should we advise for patients with knee OA?

There are two forms of exercise that can be advised. The first is aerobic exercise, which increases general fitness. This has benefits in improving well-being, helping weight loss and improving sleep pattern. Aerobic exercise also has other health benefits and is recommended in many other medical conditions. Local strengthening exercises such as quadriceps exercises improve muscle power around the knee joint and help to reduce pain and disability. Both forms of exercise are suitable for most people, albeit at different levels. If the patient is unaccustomed to exercise then the programme should be introduced gradually, working up to a level suitable for the individual patient. It is worth emphasizing that these forms of exercise should be continued regularly in the long term and not regarded as a one-off course.

4.7 How do I persuade my older patients with OA to increase their aerobic exercise?

Many patients who have not exercised for some time will automatically reject the idea of increasing activity and many will say that their knee or hip hurts too much to try. With these patients, one of the first strategies is to try to reduce their pain so that they can move more easily. Suggest a very gradual increase in activity, perhaps only walking a little further each day or week, and make sure that they return for follow-up visits to encourage motivation. Some patients who find it difficult to motivate themselves may benefit from a physiotherapy referral to instigate a graded exercise programme. In some areas it is possible to write an 'exercise prescription' where the patient attends a local leisure centre and is assessed by trained staff who can then suggest a suitable exercise programme. If you can suggest an activity that the patient will enjoy, such as social dancing, they may be more likely to persist with this activity instead of just 'doing exercise for exercise's sake'.

4.8 What is meant by 'pacing activities'?

Pacing activities means conserving energy by prioritizing tasks or activities and performing these activities at intervals during the day. Thus tasks are broken up into manageable amounts which can be spread over a period of time. This decreases the stresses put onto the joints and gives them a recovery time. At the end of the day, the same tasks have been performed but with less stress on joints and less aggravation of symptoms for the patient.

4.9 Does hormone replacement therapy have any influence on the development of OA?

There is some evidence that HRT may reduce the risk of developing OA of the hip and knee, but this is not sufficient to recommend it as a strategy unless it was being taken for some other purpose. Women who take HRT often have a feeling of well-being and may be more active, thereby possibly reducing the symptoms of OA.

4.10 Are self-help groups useful and should the primary care team refer patients to them?

Self-help groups can be very useful for many patients with OA. Groups can work in different ways. Some basically provide support to patients who all suffer from the same condition by having regular meetings to provide information and advice within a social setting. Other groups work by providing short courses, usually lasting around 6 weeks, to enable the individual patient to develop a structure for his or her own management of the condition of OA. This may be achieved by means of simple goal-setting with encouragement at each stage of the process. The hope is that, by the end of the course, the individual will have developed the resources to deal with the problems presented by the condition of OA, particularly in terms of pain management. These courses are run by OA sufferers themselves who have had special training, and the hope is that patients who find the courses useful will feel encouraged to undergo training themselves and become course leaders, thus providing more courses to deal with the ever-increasing number of OA sufferers. These courses are run and funded by Arthritis Care and are similar to the courses run for RA (see Appendix 3).

There is no specific mechanism for referral by the primary care team to self-help groups but it is important that patients are given information about the courses and the support groups, together with local contact details. They can then decide for themselves whether to self-refer.

4.11 How can we assess the impact of OA on our patients?

Some well-validated instruments are available to assess the impact of OA. WOMAC (Western Ontario and MacMaster Universities Osteoarthritis Index) is a three-dimensional scale looking at pain, stiffness and physical function in OA of hip, knee or hand. The scale is self-administered and is available in two formats: either a visual analogue scale or a Likert scale (see Appendix 1).

The second well-validated scale is the Lequesne Algofunctional Indices (see Appendix 2). There are two indices: one for hip and one for knee. This scale looks at pain, maximum distance walked and activities of daily living. It is more complex than the WOMAC scale and requires an interviewer.

Neither of these scales is suitable for a routine visit to the doctor, but may be very useful in follow-up visits and to assess the long-term impact of OA on patients. Using the 10-cm line alone for pain during a surgery consultation may give a quick idea of the patient's pain control and whether this has deteriorated since previous visits. Once a patient gets used to the

> **BOX 4.2 Factors used to assess outcome of an OA management programme**
> - Pain
> - Function
> - WOMAC or Lequesne scales
> - Body weight
> - Prescribed drug use
> - Over-the-counter (OTC) drug use

idea of filling in a questionnaire such as the WOMAC scale on regular follow-up visits, they very often like this approach to monitoring their condition and are prepared to spend the extra time it takes to fill in the forms. With elderly patients you may have to remind them to bring their glasses!

Other scales such as the HAQ (Health Assessment Questionnaire) and the SF36 (Short Form 36) are sometimes used, but these are more general scales and do not look at the impact of OA in particular.

4.12 What are the most important factors to audit in assessing any improvements in outcome following an OA management programme?

There are a number of factors that could be measured (*see Box 4.2*). However, although it is tempting to try to capture as much information as possible, it is sometimes better to concentrate on auditing just one or two outcomes.

EDUCATIONAL ISSUES

4.13 What is the place of patient education in OA and how should this be achieved?

Patient education is one of the most important tools we have in the management of OA. A patient who understands the background of OA, the various lifestyle factors affecting the outcome, the large number of drug and non-drug interventions and the likely prognosis is much better equipped to manage his or her own condition with input from various health professionals as required. Although in the past patients have been poorly informed about their medical problems, the climate is changing and management of long-term conditions such as OA is now seen as a partnership between patient and health professionals. It is our duty as doctors, nurses and therapists to provide education ideally at every patient contact, although given the time pressure on appointments this is not easy to do in primary care.

GPs, however, do have the advantage of seeing patients at intervals over long periods of time and each contact can be used to provide information or reinforce previous messages. Physiotherapists now see education as a pivotal part of their job and many practice nurses spend much of their time in patient education.

When an initial diagnosis of OA is given to the patient, the doctor needs to take some time to explain the nature and likely outcome of the condition. Many patients just hear the word 'arthritis' and imagine their future to be one of severe disability, perhaps in a wheelchair. Written information such as the Primary Care Rheumatology Society leaflet on knee OA or the Arthritis Research Campaign leaflets on OA and knee OA are useful at this stage. A follow-up visit is advised, either with the doctor or with the practice nurse if appropriate, to reinforce educational and lifestyle measures and to answer the patient's questions once they have had time to reflect and digest the information. The newly formed website Move (*see Appendix 3*) is a source of information for patients with OA and also for the primary care team and specialists.

Education of the public at large is also important. Many people still regard OA as inevitable with increasing age and assume that nothing can be done to prevent or slow down the problem. Maintenance of a normal weight and regular suitable exercise are important at all ages and these important health messages fit well with the type of healthier lifestyle we advocate for a large number of medical conditions such as coronary artery disease, diabetes and osteoporosis.

4.14 How can we change the negative image of OA within the medical and nursing communities?

Many health professionals still regard OA as inevitable with increasing age and have a pessimistic attitude to treatment and outcome. Much of this attitude relates to training and it is important that those responsible for teaching health professionals are aware of the modern approach to OA in terms of non-pharmacological as well as pharmacological management. Patients with joint pains should be encouraged to discuss their problems with a suitably trained health professional and to receive lifestyle advice to try to prevent progression of the condition. Encouragement of weight loss and increased exercise would have major benefits not only in terms of OA but also in the prevention of other conditions such as osteoporosis, heart disease and diabetes. The promotion of a healthier lifestyle is often the remit of practice nurses, many of whom are unaware of the benefits to joints which may result.

BOX 4.3 Topics to be included in a patient education plan

■ The nature of OA
■ The likely prognosis
■ Strategies for dealing with pain
■ Written information in the form of leaflets, videos and website addresses
■ Advice on self-management
■ Advice on simple analgesia
■ Support group information, including OA-specific websites (e.g. Move; *see Appendix 3*)

4.15 What should be included in a patient education plan?

The aspects listed in Box 4.3 should be included.

4.16 What support groups are there for patients with OA?

Arthritis Care runs support groups around the country. In the past there has been a perception that these groups catered more for patients with inflammatory arthritis than for those with OA. These attitudes are changing as OA is recognized as a major cause of disability, and many patients with OA find enormous benefit from attending a group where they can meet fellow sufferers and give each other support. Arthritis Care also runs self-management programmes; patients attend for a 6-week course and are taught to manage their own condition and develop strategies for coping with pain and disability. All these courses are run by people who suffer from OA themselves and patients derive enormous benefit from them.

ENVIRONMENTAL ISSUES

4.17 What factors should be considered within doctors' premises to accommodate patients with moderate to severe OA?

From 2003 all public premises should, by law, have access and toilet facilities for the disabled. This should include wheelchair access and ramps. Many patients who do not fall into the category of 'disabled' nevertheless benefit from some thought being given to surgery facilities. Patients with knee and hip OA, as well as patients with back pain, find that modern low seating is difficult to use; higher seating, preferably with arms to help the patient push up into the standing position, is much more 'patient-friendly'. Many patients need handrails when negotiating steps, and grab rails at doors and in toilets. Steps and low stools are useful when getting on and off examination couches.

4.18 With the ageing population, many more people have OA. What environmental and behavioural changes are required within society to cope with this problem?

The first priority is to raise awareness of the condition of OA and all the difficulties that it presents. Things are slowly changing. In the UK there is a greater move towards ensuring that facilities for the disabled are present within all public buildings, including health care units such as hospitals and doctors' and dentists' surgeries.

Good access to buildings is essential but is in itself not much use if patients have difficulty getting there. Many disabled patients find great difficulty with public transport and, unless they can afford taxis, have to rely on friends or relatives to give them lifts, which may be logistically difficult due to distance or time pressures. Many people do not wish to be a burden and so stop asking for help and gradually become increasingly socially isolated. Some areas of the country have buses with low walk-on platforms or platforms that descend as required; other areas run 'dial-a-bus' services where an individual who is registered with the scheme can phone for a bus to pick them up at home and go to various specified local facilities. Many local areas run voluntary services providing transport to GPs' surgeries or hospitals, both for outpatient appointments and for visiting.

Social services such as home helps, meals on wheels, neck alarms, lunch clubs and day centres play a large part in enabling elderly arthritic patients to continue to live in their own homes, although in many parts of the country these facilities may be difficult to access.

4.19 Who should be responsible for co-ordinating care for people with OA within the community?

GPs are potentially best placed to co-ordinate care for people with OA within the community as they have access to all the various players who can provide help and care (*see Box 4.4*).

BOX 4.4 Providers of help and care within the community for OA sufferers

- Community-based staff, such as district nurses and health visitors
- Therapists, such as physiotherapists and occupational therapists
- Social services
- Benefits agencies
- Pharmacists
- Dieticians
- Self-help groups

Non-pharmacological management 2: Physical therapies and complementary therapies

5

PQ PATIENT QUESTIONS

PHYSICAL THERAPIES

5.1 What are the most useful aids and appliances to assist a patient disabled by OA to remain independent at home?

There are many useful aids and appliances (*see Box 5.1*) and their suitability will depend on the individual requirements of the patient. An occupational therapist is the best person to advise on the most appropriate aids, although many patients choose simple aids from catalogues. *See also Q. 5.27.*

5.2 A patient with knee OA wishes to exercise and swim at his local leisure centre. He comes to ask your advice about which exercises would be best and which should be avoided. How would you advise him?

Exercises that involve direct impact such as running on a treadmill are probably best avoided. Aerobic exercise can be effectively achieved by using a cross-trainer or a ski machine; here there is no direct impact, as the foot remains in contact with the pedal or ski at all times. Many gyms will have equipment that is designed to provide resistance to certain muscle groups, and this can be effectively used to strengthen quadriceps. Static cycling is also useful as the body weight is supported while the leg muscles are exercised, although it is important to make sure that the saddle is at the correct height to avoid too much pressure on a bent knee.

In general, swimming is fine for knee OA although the kick of breaststroke may aggravate knee pain by producing sideways stresses.

For all exercises, it is important to advise the patient to build up gradually and to stop any exercises that produce an exacerbation of symptoms. In some cases, however, although initial exercise produces some discomfort, this will ease as muscle strength builds up and exercise may become completely pain free. *See also Q. 5.26.*

5.3 What advice could you give a keen gardener with knee OA who finds kneeling for even a short time extremely painful?

First of all it might be worth trying knee pads, a kneeling mat or a stool while gardening although all these still require bent knees. Long-handled tools such as forks, hoes and rakes can be used while standing upright. In the longer term it may be helpful to change the garden layout to incorporate raised beds, which are easier to maintain with less bending, and to change the planting to make more use of shrubs and perennials together with ground-cover plants to minimize weeding and short-term planting.

BOX 5.1　Available aids to assist independence at home

■ Transfer aids help transfer the patient from sitting to standing. Patients with hip and knee OA can sometimes manage to walk once they are in the upright position but are unable to stand by themselves without help. Transfer aids include higher more upright seats, power-lift or spring-loaded armchairs which propel the patient from sitting to standing and simple armrests and rails.

■ Walking aids provide support, and include walking sticks, tripods and wheeled aids.

■ Transport aids, such as wheelchairs, can be either self- or attendant-propelled.

■ Stair-lifts for transferring from floor to floor within the house may be essential for enabling a patient to remain in his or her own home.

■ Toilet aids include raised toilet seats, toilet frames and handles at the side of the toilet for support.

■ Bathing aids include lifts or hoists, seats within the bath or shower, non-slip mats and grab handles.

■ Feeding aids include two-handled cups and large-handled cutlery.

■ Dressing aids include use of Velcro instead of buttons or laces, long-handled shoehorns and stocking aids.

■ Hygiene aids include long-handled brushes for grooming and teeth-cleaning, electric toothbrush and tap levers.

■ Communication aids include remote door-opener, speaker phones and preset telephone numbers.

■ Housework aids include potholders, sponges instead of cloths, specially designed scissors and machines to reduce effort, such as blenders, food processors and electric can-openers.

■ Recreational aids include remote controls for televisions and other equipment, book-holders and long-handled reachers for picking up at a distance.

5.4　Can too much exercise damage joints?

It is probably true that too much exercise of a certain kind can cause joint damage. On the whole, however, this applies to overuse such as in elite athletics, football, etc., where the joint is subject to severe strains. There is no evidence that leisure exercise such as jogging causes joint damage, although it may exacerbate symptoms in a joint already affected by OA. Moderate exercise is good for joints and should be encouraged.

> A recent study (Sutton et al 2001) found no evidence to suggest that increased levels of regular physical activity throughout life lead to an increased risk of knee OA in later life. There was, however, an increased risk of OA if there was a history of previous knee injury. As most knee injuries are associated with sporting activity, it is important to consider the type of sporting activity, as some sports are much more likely to cause knee injury than others. Higher-risk sports include football, rugby, ski-ing, squash and weight-lifting.

5.5 Is it sensible for a patient with knee OA to use a knee support while exercising?

When a patient with knee OA starts on a weight-bearing exercise programme it may be helpful to use a support at this stage. Later, however, it is best not to use a support so that the muscles can build up strength and so provide more support to the joint in the long term. If the patient finds that it is too uncomfortable to exercise without using a support then it is better to continue using it rather than stop the patient exercising at all. The support should be used for the specific exercise, not all the time.

5.6 Should all patients with a new diagnosis of OA be seen by a physiotherapist?

Ideally, all patients with a new diagnosis of OA should be seen and assessed by a physiotherapist to advise about appropriate exercise, joint protection and muscle-strengthening exercises depending on the joints involved (Hurley & Scott 1998). If all OA patients were given the benefit of an early physiotherapy consultation concentrating on education and self-management, this would most likely result in improved outcomes and less dependence on drug therapy and the medical model of care. Such a scheme is unlikely to happen at present due to shortage of physiotherapists and long waiting times for treatment, but if it were possible it would most probably be cost-effective in the long term.

Patients can of course be shown suitable exercises and joint protection at a surgery consultation, although this is unlikely to be as in-depth or as personal as a physiotherapy consultation. In this situation printed leaflets are very useful, especially those showing muscle-strengthening exercises for individual joints such as quadriceps exercises for knee OA. Both the Arthritis Research Campaign and the Primary Care Rheumatology Society provide leaflets on knee OA (*see Appendix 3*).

5.7 What is the purpose of physiotherapy referral for patients with OA?

Modern physiotherapy aims not only to assess and treat patients with

---

BOX 5.2 Advice on exercise from the physiotherapist

- When to rest and when to exercise
- How to pace activities to spread the load over a period of time
- Posture if appropriate
- How to protect joints and how to reduce stress on particular joints
- Muscle-building exercises to protect joints

BOX 5.3 Treatments available from the physiotherapist

- Heat and cold
- Exercise regime
- Strapping
- Knee brace
- Conditioning programmes using swimming or hydrotherapy
- Gait analysis
- Biomechanical assessment of feet, which may result in the use of heel wedges or arch supports
- TENS (transcutaneous electrical nerve stimulation)
- Acupuncture
- Some physiotherapists have a qualification in injection techniques and may offer them.

---

musculoskeletal problems but also to educate patients about their condition and advise on exercise programmes designed to address problems on an individual basis (*see Box 5.2*).

As well as playing an advisory role the physiotherapist may instigate some treatments (*see Box 5.3*).

5.8   When should splinting be used in OA?

One joint that responds well to splinting is the first carpometacarpal joint of the thumb. A resting splint, often worn at night, can be very effective in helping to relieve pain. Knee braces are sometimes used to correct biomechanical abnormalities that put unequal stresses on to the joint. These braces fit around the thigh and upper calf and are joined together by hinge mechanisms which are often quite sophisticated and provide balancing pressure at various levels to correct the underlying abnormality.

5.9   What is meant by patellar taping?

If the patient is suffering from patellofemoral OA, it is worth trying patellar taping to relieve pain (Cushnaghan et al 1994). The patella is taped medially to alter the glide of the patella on the underlying structures. To apply this technique, the knee is first taped with two pieces of stretch tape totally covering the patella (*see Fig. 5.1a*). A particular type of tensioning tape is then applied onto this stretch tape at the lateral border of the patella. This is then pulled medially and the tape is fixed at the medial border at the medial femoral condyle (*see Fig. 5.1b*). The positioning may need to be adjusted for each individual patient to gain the best relief of pain (*see Fig. 5.1c*).

5.10   Is TENS useful in OA and what is the rationale underlying its use?

TENS stands for transcutaneous electrical nerve stimulation. Machines for delivering TENS are usually battery-operated and small enough to fit in a pocket. The device generates an electrical waveform which is transmitted to the skin via small electrode pads.

The rationale for the use of TENS is explained by the 'gate' theory of pain. Small diameter nerve fibres carry pain stimuli through a 'gate mechanism'; impulses carried by larger diameter nerve fibres going through the same 'gate' can inhibit transmission of impulses by the smaller nerves. TENS stimulates the nerve fibres of larger diameter, effectively closing the 'gate' to the smaller fibres which would normally transmit the sensation of pain to the higher centres.

Most TENS machines can produce a range of pulse widths and variable rates of stimulation and it is worth experimenting with different settings to find which gives the individual patient the best pain relief. Most patients find that a frequency in the range of 50–100 Hz is most effective and generally, at this range, patients experience a pleasant tingling sensation. If TENS produces some pain relief the patient often finds that they can then begin to move the affected muscles and this then brings about an improvement in the general condition. Some patients seem to gain long-

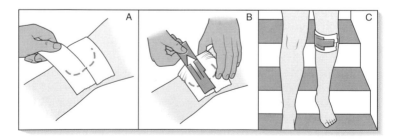

▲

Fig. 5.1 Patellar taping (see text for explanation of the technique). Courtesy of BSN Medical.

lasting benefit from TENS whereas others find it of no use at all. Many pain clinics and physiotherapy departments and, indeed GPs' surgeries, are willing to lend TENS machines for a short time to allow patients to find whether this therapy is effective for them. If it is, they can then purchase one for themselves. TENS is very safe and is self-administered and is a very useful option for some patients.

5.11 What is the most suitable footwear for a patient with lower-limb OA?

The impact of repeated heel strikes on a surface produces jarring which is then transmitted through the joints of the lower limb, often causing irritation and a deterioration in symptoms. This jarring can be reduced by the use of something to absorb impact, such as an impact-absorbing insole in an ordinary shoe or a specially designed shoe with built-in impact absorption. Although there are specialist shoes available, the cheapest solution is a good training shoe with a suitably thick sole. As well as having an impact-absorbing sole, a suitable shoe should also be flat, have a broad forefoot and a soft upper and have secure fastenings (i.e. not slip-ons).

5.12 How can heel wedges help patients with OA knee?

Knee OA can produce a varus deformity at the knee. Sometimes a heel wedge placed within the shoe can correct this deformity and may bring considerable relief of symptoms. Heel wedges are cheap, simple and safe and are well worth trying. If correcting the deformity produces no benefit it is sometimes worth trying the wedge at the other side of the shoe. At a recent EULAR conference, a poster presentation on heel wedges demonstrated reduction in NSAID (non-steroidal anti-inflammatory drug) usage.

5.13 Is it worthwhile giving sorbothane arch supports for patients with OA knee?

If the patient has a fallen arch this can alter the biomechanics within the lower limb. An arch support may be sufficient to correct this and to reduce symptoms and can be a cheap, safe and effective form of therapy.

5.14 Are patients with hypermobility at greater risk of OA?

Hypermobility (double-jointedness) allows a joint to move beyond its normal range and may lead to OA by causing abnormal stresses on the joint over a period of time. Classically, patients can be diagnosed as having hypermobility if they fulfil certain criteria, including scoring

TABLE 5.1 The Beighton Score

Classic signs of hypermobility	Points (total points 9)		
	Right	Right and left	Left
Dorsiflexion of the fifth metacarpophalangeal to 90°	1		1
Apposition of thumb to volar aspect of forearm	1		1
Hyperextension of the elbow by 10°	1		1
Hyperextension of the knee by 10°	1		1
Hands flat on the floor with knees extended		1	

4 out of 9 points on the Beighton Score (*see Table 5.1*) and having arthralgia for 3 months or more in three or more different joints. If a patient is diagnosed as having hypermobility, they should be educated in care of the joints with a muscle-strengthening programme to avoid overstretching the joint capsule and surrounding structures. They should also have specialized advice about warming up before taking exercise and, equally importantly, warming down, to allow stretched tendons to return slowly to their normal tension. The Arthritis Research Campaign leaflet on hypermobility is very informative.

5.15 What help can an occupational therapist give to a patient with OA?

The purpose of occupational therapy is to provide aids and appliances to enable a patient to function better and to assist the patient in being as independent as possible while performing the functions of daily living (*see Box 5.1*).

As well as functional aids for daily living, there are many useful and imaginative aids available to enable patients to try to continue hobbies and leisure activities despite their handicap. For example, there are racks for holding books and others for holding playing cards, as well as specialist aids for recreational activities such as fishing, gardening and bowling (*see Fig. 5.2*).

COMPLEMENTARY THERAPIES

5.16 What is the place of complementary therapy in the management of OA?

 Patients who develop chronic painful diseases with no apparent cure often turn to alternative therapies. Some may have found no benefit from

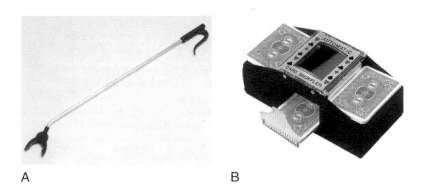

A   B

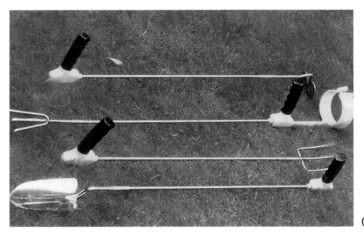

C

▲

Fig. 5.2 Aids for reaching (a), shuffling cards (b) and (c) gardening are designed to allow patients to continue the hobbies and leisure activities they enjoy despite their osteoarthritis. Courtesy of Homecraft.

conventional management, some may have experienced side-effects from drugs such as anti-inflammatories and some may prefer not to take drug therapy at all. Most of these complementary therapies do not have any evidence base to back up their claims of benefit although there is no doubt that many patients find these therapies effective. Increasingly, conventional randomized controlled studies are being set up to try to assess the benefits of these treatments. Several meta-analyses (Ezzo et al 2001, Long & Ernst 2001) have been performed looking at past studies in homeopathy and acupuncture, but these have not produced any substantial evidence. Some reasons for the benefits found by patients on taking complementary therapies may include those listed in Box 5.4.

A small but increasing number of GPs use alternative therapies in their NHS surgeries, but for most patients these therapies are not available on the NHS. Recently, however, some projects have been put in place to support the setting up of integrated complementary services within primary care trusts and, if successful, these should increase the availability and accessibility of such treatments.

A recent survey of patients attending rheumatology and orthopaedic outpatient departments showed that more than a quarter had already used some form of complementary therapy and, of these, around half said that they had gained some benefit.

5.17 Is there any regulation of practitioners offering complementary therapies?

Some branches of complementary therapy now have statutory regulations following the formation of the General Osteopathic Council and the

---

BOX 5.4 Possible reasons for the benefits to patients of complementary therapies

- The increased time given to patients by complementary practitioners compared with time available in the increasingly under-resourced and overstretched NHS, both in primary and secondary care.
- Although some areas have access to complementary therapy provided by the NHS, most areas do not and here the patients have to pay for treatment. Treatment is often valued more when it has to be paid for!
- Complementary therapies are mostly drug-free and this is appealing to many patients.
- Many complementary therapists are good at evaluating the 'whole person'. This holistic approach is one frequently used by GPs, but time pressures often prevent optimum benefit being obtained.

General Chiropractic Council. Some alternative practitioners, however, have variable professional training, are not members of any professional body and do not have to swear the Hippocratic Oath. Although planned, there is at present no statutory legislation in the UK covering those who offer acupuncture treatment. There are, however, three professional societies for acupuncturists, including the British Medical Acupuncture Society, the British Acupuncture Council and the Acupuncture Association of Chartered Physiotherapists.

5.18 What forms of complementary therapy are available for patients with OA?

Homeopathy, herbal medicine and nutritional therapies act as alternatives to the pharmacological approaches of conventional medicine. Osteopathy, chiropractic techniques and acupuncture are used instead of the conventional biomechanical approaches of physiotherapy and surgery, while hypnotherapy, reflexology, relaxation techniques and various other sensory therapies replace the more conventional approaches of patient education and clinical psychology.

5.19 Is there any evidence that acupuncture is effective in OA?

Acupuncture is used by a number of complementary therapists and also increasingly by physiotherapists. A recent meta-analysis of acupuncture for OA of the knee (Ezzo et al 2001) suggested that there was limited evidence for acupuncture being more effective than being wait-listed for treatment or having usual treatment, in terms of pain and function. For pain, there was some evidence that real acupuncture was more effective than sham acupuncture. Although no definitive conclusions could be drawn and further controlled trials are required, the authors suggest that acupuncture may have a place in the treatment of knee OA. Some large studies are at present planned both in Britain and the USA looking at acupuncture and OA, and further evidence should be available in due course.

5.20 Is there any evidence that homeopathy is effective in OA?

To date there is little good evidence for the efficacy of homeopathy in the management of OA. Long & Ernst (2001) published a review of four randomized controlled trials in homeopathy for the treatment of OA. They were unable to draw any firm conclusions for the effectiveness of homeopathic treatment in OA. One of the difficulties in performing trials of homeopathic remedies is that, in randomized controlled trials, the medication has to be standardized, whereas in normal homeopathic management the treatment is specific for the individual patient.

5.21 Can conventional and alternative therapies be used in conjunction with each other?

There is generally no reason why these therapies should not be used together. If you are treating a patient for OA with conventional therapies, it is useful to know what other therapies the patient may be using. Many patients will come and ask advice as to whether they should try complementary treatments.

5.22 Should we be encouraging or discouraging our patients to try complementary therapies?

It is difficult for those of us practising conventional medicine to actively promote complementary therapies in view of the lack of evidence supporting their use. On the other hand, many patients seem to derive some benefit from such therapies, at least in the short term, and it could be argued that we do not have the right to discourage our patients from trying potentially useful treatments. Personally, I neither encourage nor discourage my patients from trying these therapies if they wish to. Most therapies will do no harm and may do some good, and if patients find no benefit they will discontinue the therapy of their own accord. In some conditions such as RA, it is important that patients who are attending complementary therapists do not discontinue their conventional medication such as DMARDs (disease-modifying anti-rheumatic drugs). In OA, however, this does not apply and the main potential loss to patients of stopping their conventional therapy might be loss of symptom control.

5.23 Are herbal medicines useful in OA and, if so, which ones should be tried?

The meta-analysis by Long et al (2001) suggested that there was some evidence for the efficacy of some herbal medicines in OA. Herbal products for which there was some weak evidence in the form of single randomized controlled trials included Rheumalex, willow bark, common stinging nettle and Articulin-F. Those with two favourable trials included devil's claw and extract of avocado and soya bean, otherwise known as avocado/soybean unsaponifiables; those with three or more favourable trials included Phytodolor. These herbal products appear to be fairly safe, with a low incidence of side-effects, and may produce benefits for individual patients. As with all complementary therapies, more research needs to be undertaken with herbal medicines to ascertain their true effectiveness.

BOX 5.5 Possible side-effects of some alternative therapies

■ Chiropractic or osteopathic manipulation of the neck may rarely cause damage to the carotid artery leading to stroke.

■ Acupuncture needles must be sterile to avoid transfer of diseases such as hepatitis B and C and HIV.

■ Acupuncture needles can very occasionally damage blood vessels, lungs and nerves.

■ Devil's claw, a herbal medicine recommended for relief of pain in OA, may interact with conventional medicines such as warfarin and hypoglycaemic and beta-blocking drugs. This product may also cause problems in patients who have a history of peptic ulceration or gallstones.

5.24   Are there any serious side-effects of complementary or alternative therapies?

Although alternative therapies are perceived to be safe, some of them can occasionally cause side-effects (*see Box 5.5*) and patients wishing to try alternative therapies should be advised to find a practitioner with some professional qualifications.

5.25   Is there any evidence for the effectiveness of copper or magnetic bracelets in OA?

The Arthritis Research Campaign is at present funding a study looking at the value of magnetic bracelets in OA, so hopefully we will have some definitive answers in due course. Copper bracelets have traditionally been used for arthritis over many years but I am not aware of any evidence supporting their use.

PQ PATIENT QUESTIONS

5.26   I have OA of my knees. What exercises are helpful and what may be harmful for this?

There are certain specific exercises, such as quadriceps-strengthening exercises, which will increase the muscle strength around the knee joint and help to protect it from external stresses. These exercises can be taught by a physiotherapist or you can find a description of how to do the exercises in leaflets on OA of the knee from the Arthritis Research Campaign and Primary Care Rheumatology Society (*see Appendix 3*).

PQ PATIENT QUESTIONS

If you can strengthen your knee in this way, you should find that other exercise is easier and less painful. Cycling is a suitable exercise for knee OA, although you should be careful to have the seat height adjusted so that you do not put too much stress on a partly bent knee. Brisk walking is an excellent exercise, although you should try to use footwear that has impact-absorbing soles, especially if you are walking on hard pavements. Swimming is generally good exercise, although the kick of breaststroke may aggravate symptoms from knee OA. Backstroke and crawl are usually fine. Exercise involving stepping or walking on rough ground may cause a flare of pain and stiffness in the knee.

5.27 I have heard that there are various aids to help people with arthritis. How can I find out about these?

Several large companies produce catalogues of products designed to help people with arthritis. The occupational therapy department of your local hospital would probably be able to give you some contact details of local suppliers. Arthritis Care also has information available (*see Appendix 3*). Yellow Pages may help, and some of the larger pharmacies have very comprehensive catalogues.

5.28 My doctor referred me for a course of physiotherapy for my OA but when I went they did not give me any specific treatment but merely showed me some exercises to do. I was very disappointed, as I was expecting something to help with the pain and all this does is make it worse.

Much of a physiotherapist's work is concerned with showing patients how to help themselves in the form of exercises to do to strengthen various muscles. They may also advise on specific aids such as walking sticks and heel inserts and taping of the kneecap. Sometimes physiotherapists use heat and cold treatments, manipulation, ultrasound and TENS treatments, but these may only be suitable in certain conditions and presumably in your case the physiotherapist did not feel that any of these treatments were appropriate. Sometimes when you start to do exercises that you have not been used to doing you can find that your muscles become sore and stiff. This is a normal response, but usually it wears off as you gradually increase the exercise. If the exercises are aggravating your pain, then it is worth speaking to your physiotherapist. Perhaps the exercises are not best suited for your particular circumstances, perhaps you are not doing them correctly or perhaps you have tried to build up your exercise programme too quickly.

5.29 I have a painful knee due to OA. My doctor suggested that I should try a stick. Should I use this stick on the affected side or the good side?

A walking stick can be very useful in OA of the knee as it helps to reduce the pressure on the affected knee by up to 50%. You should use the stick on the 'good' side. Ask a physiotherapist or occupational therapist to assess you for a stick to ensure that it is the correct height.

5.30   How do I check to see if the stick my friend gave to me is the correct length?

It is not complicated to do this with a little help from a friend. Stand straight with your arm by your side and the stick should come to the 'crease' of your wrist. You will need to cut any excess length off the bottom and replace the ferrule if it is worn. If the stick does not come up to the wrist crease then you will have to find a longer stick!

5.31   I have painful and stiff hips and knees due to OA. I am finding it increasingly difficult to use the toilet and have to pull myself up using the towel rail. Is there anything that will help?

Ask your doctor or physiotherapist to refer you to an occupational therapist who can assess you for a raised toilet seat. This should mean that you do not have to bend as far down to use the toilet and straightening up again should be much easier. A handle fixed to the wall beside the toilet would also give you support and make it easier for you to pull yourself up.

5.32   One of my friends finds that using an ice pack on her knee helps to relieve the pain of her arthritis. I would have thought that using a heat pack or hot water bottle would be much more comforting.

You are both correct; while some people find cold more useful to relieve pain and stiffness, others find that warmth is better. There is no right or wrong, and whatever you find most helpful is what you should use. If you are using cold in the form of an ice pack or bag of frozen peas remember to wrap it to avoid direct contact with the skin. Similarly, heat packs and hot water bottles should also be wrapped to avoid burning the skin.

5.33   My doctor has suggested that I should wear trainers to protect my knees which have OA. Although I find trainers comfortable I think they look ugly. Are there any alternatives?

An ideal shoe for those people with OA of their hips and knees should be flat, have a thick sole which can absorb impact, have soft uppers and a broad forefoot. Trainers usually fulfil all these requirements but are not the only answer. Some fashion shoes are made with impact-absorbing soles and the other essential features described above. Several manufacturers now produce such shoes, which come in a variety of styles and colours; most good shoe shops should be able to advise you. If you still do not like these shoes, another option is to wear an impact-absorbing insole made of a thin material such as sorbothane inside your own fashion shoes. This will give a degree of protection although it is not ideal.

5.34 My physiotherapist suggested that I should try a TENS machine for the pain of my OA knee. I am a bit afraid to use it as I believe it produces an electrical current through the skin. Does this have any side-effects?

No. TENS is remarkably free from side-effects. When you use it you normally feel a tingling sensation which can be lessened or increased as you wish, to get the best result for you. This tingling is just part of the way TENS works and it will do you no harm. TENS is not effective for everyone but if it does work for you it is a safe and drug-free way of controlling pain and is certainly worth trying (*see Q. 5.10*).

5.35 I am tired of swallowing pills for my arthritis. Would acupuncture help?

It is certainly worthwhile trying complementary therapies as well as your doctor's medication. The principle is to find out if they can help relieve some of the pain and discomfort. Some patients find complementary therapies very effective and often a patient may be able to reduce the number of tablets they take; the extremely lucky ones will be able to reduce them to zero.

It is certainly reasonable to try acupuncture for your OA, although there is no guarantee that it will work for you. Some people do seem to get some short-term relief of symptoms with acupuncture and there are few side-effects of this treatment.

Remember that there is a range of complementary therapies such as acupuncture, reflexology and aromatherapy. Initially, try a course of three sessions and then assess if the therapy is effective. It is advisable to go to someone with certificates of competence and professional insurance, even though it is not a legal requirement for people to have professional qualifications in order to practise many of the complementary therapies. Be wary when therapists suggest that you should stop all the medications prescribed by your doctor. This could be counter-productive and even dangerous. Remember that the doctor's medications do not interfere with complementary medicines or therapies.

5.36 I have heard that some drugs given for OA can have very serious side-effects and I would like to avoid these as much as possible. Are there any herbal or homeopathic products that might help?

There is really very little evidence that herbal or homeopathic products are effective in relieving the symptoms of OA. On the other hand, there seem to be very few side-effects of such treatments and they may work for you. As with all complementary therapies, it is important that you seek advice from a suitably qualified therapist. Remember also that, while drugs in this country have to go through very strict testing before they can be used, these controls do not apply to herbal or 'natural' products.

5.37   Are there any foods that will make my arthritis worse?

It is important to eat a healthy diet in order to give you energy to exercise and to maintain a normal weight, but there is no evidence that any particular foods either worsen or improve OA. Some people feel better in general when they stick to a particular diet such as vegetarian, but this has not been shown to have any effect on OA.

5.38   Are there any foods that can improve my OA?

No specific foods have been shown to have a beneficial effect on OA, but there is a little evidence that good nutrition, especially with vitamins C and D, may prevent progression of OA.

5.39   Is it true that olive oil will lubricate my joints?

Although it is an attractive idea to think that olive oil taken by mouth will get into the joints and act as a lubricant, this does not actually happen. Olive oil, like fish oils, if taken by mouth, load an enzyme system in the body so that more anti-inflammatory proteins are made. This may well have a beneficial effect on the joints. A simple way of considering the effect is to think of these oils as having been converted into NSAIDs that the body makes naturally but without the stomach side-effects of taking NSAID tablets.

5.40   Can I buy anything from the health food shop to make my arthritis better?

It is certainly worthwhile considering some products such as:

- Glucosamine
- Olive oil
- Fish oil

Always try these products for a few weeks. If your symptoms improve, that's good, but is might be worth carrying out your own self trial: take the product for 3 weeks, then stop the tablets and see if your joints become more painful, then start the tablets again and see if they work again. This way you will only be spending money if you are sure that they work on you.

5.41   I have severe pain from my arthritis and, no matter what my doctor gives me, it doesn't help. What should I do?

This is a difficult situation and you certainly should discuss it with your doctor. Maybe the way forward is to be referred to a specialist in arthritis; sometimes referral to a pain clinic can help.

   An alternative is to seek out a local self-help group (your local library will be able to help). These can be amazingly well organized but tend to be friendly and informal. They are a good source of information and help about diseases and self-management, which often gives patients more self-belief and understanding; this helps reduce stress, which, in turn, often results in a reduction in pain. (Useful address: Arthritis Care Helpline—*see Appendix 3.*)

5.42   I would like to learn to cope with my arthritis by myself. Are there any books or courses available?

The Arthritis Research Campaign produces a long list of informative booklets dealing with different aspects of OA. These include not only information about OA itself and how it may affect different joints but also information about such things as footwear, seating and activities. For a full list of leaflets contact the Arthritis Research Campaign (*see Appendix 3*).

Arthritis Care runs support groups around the country and also runs self-management programmes which teach participants to deal with their own condition in terms of pain and mobility (*see Appendix 3*).

Pharmacological management 1: Topical treatments

6

6.1 Which patients benefit from topical treatments?

Many patients find topical treatments soothing and seem to experience relief of symptoms by using them. Also, many patients do not like to take oral drug therapy at all and others who are already taking other essential medication prefer not to add to their oral drug intake. For all these patients, a trial of topical treatment is useful. All topical preparations have another advantage in that the patient becomes directly involved in his or her own care by actually having to apply the cream or ointment two to four times daily. This can sit well with a management plan where the patient is directly involved in setting up and continuing a self-efficacy programme rather than sitting back and waiting for a drug to have an effect.

Topical preparations are not indicated for severe symptoms as they are usually only effective in mild to moderate OA, but they may be added as concomitant therapy perhaps to analgesics before moving on to oral NSAIDs (non-steroidal anti-inflammatory drugs). As indicated elsewhere, oral medications can have significant side-effects. Analgesics can cause constipation and central nervous system side-effects, particularly in elderly patients; NSAIDs can cause major adverse effects, particularly in the gastrointestinal tract. These adverse events not only result in around 2000 deaths per year but also result in a five times increased relative risk of hospitalization due to a gastrointestinal complication compared with the general population.

There are a number of different topical preparations, including:

- Rubefacients
- Topical NSAIDs
- Capsaicin.

There is no real evidence to support the use of rubefacients, but they have been available for many years, are cheap and have no real side-effects.

Topical NSAIDs are not popular with prescribing advisors who feel that there is insufficient evidence to support the use of these relatively expensive agents. However, there is some evidence to suggest that some patients do benefit from topical NSAIDs. A meta-analysis (Moore et al 1998) showed that, in chronic pain conditions such as OA, topical NSAIDs were significantly better than placebo over 2 weeks with a number needed to treat of 3.1. To date there have been no large-scale studies comparing oral and topical NSAIDs. There is no doubt that the risk of developing the serious side-effects of oral NSAIDs is vastly reduced with topical therapy. If a patient finds a topical NSAID beneficial and if it results in not prescribing analgesics and NSAIDs, this may actually be cost-effective as not only are there savings in not prescribing oral drugs but there are also savings in not prescribing other drugs to treat side-effects such as constipation with

analgesics or prophylaxis to prevent gastrointestinal problems with oral NSAIDs.
There is some doubt as to the exact mechanism of action of topical NSAIDs. Some think that it is mainly the act of rubbing or massage that is effective, although there are data showing that drug levels within the joint indicate that there is direct absorption through the skin and that this is what accounts for the efficacy. Many topical NSAIDs can be bought in the pharmacy without a prescription, and patients can be advised to try some different preparations to see whether they find them effective. Those available over the counter include ibuprofen, piroxicam, ketoprofen and felbinac.

6.2 What is the place of a topical formulation in the management of OA?

Most guidelines for the management of OA suggest that lifestyle and physical features should be addressed first. If pharmacological therapy is required then simple analgesics such as paracetamol should be used as a first line. If this does not relieve pain, then before moving on to stronger analgesics or to oral NSAIDs it is sensible to try a topical therapy. Some patients will find considerable benefit from such formulations and may never require stronger remedies if their OA remains mild. For others with slowly progressing symptoms, the use of topical therapies may delay the time when they will require to move up the analgesic ladder. For others, however, topical therapies will provide no help with symptoms and they will require oral therapies of stronger analgesics or oral NSAIDs.

6.3 Which topical medication can be prescribed with NSAIDs and COX-2 inhibitors?

Rubefacients and capsaicin can be prescribed together with NSAIDs and COX-2 (cyclo-oxygenase-2) inhibitors, but topical NSAIDs should not be prescribed with these treatments.

6.4 Which topical medication can be prescribed with analgesics?

Rubefacients, capsaicin cream and topical NSAIDs can all be prescribed together with analgesics.

6.5 Is capsicum, found in rubefacients, the same as capsaicin?

No. Capsicum and capsaicin are different and work in different ways, although both are applied topically. Capsicum is an ingredient found in rubefacients which, on rubbing onto the skin, gives a feeling of warmth and vasodilatation. Capsaicin, on the other hand, is derived from hot chillies and is thought to exert its action by entering the joint and depleting substance P, which is a neuropeptide involved in the transmission of pain in the afferent fibres.

6.6 How does topical capsaicin relieve pain in OA joints?

Joints that are inflamed have raised levels of substance P, which is a neuropeptide involved in the transmission of pain in the afferent nerve fibres. Substance P is thought to stimulate synoviocytes to produce prostaglandins and collagenases, leading to inflammation. Repeated topical use of capsaicin is thought to gradually deplete the amount of substance P within the joint, thus interfering with pain transmission to the higher centres. In order to reduce substance P levels it is important to apply the capsaicin cream regularly as a very small bead four times a day for around 4 weeks before maximum benefit is attained.

Capsaicin is very safe. The only real side-effect is that of burning or tingling on application, which is experienced by around half of all patients, but this generally settles within the first few weeks. It is important to wash hands after use to avoid contact with sensitive body areas such as the eyes.

Capsaicin cream is only available on prescription. Both the American College of Rheumatology (Hochberg et al 1995) and the Primary Care Rheumatology Society, in their respective guidelines for the management of OA of the knee, suggest use of capsaicin and other topical agents as coming after a trial of paracetamol but before use of oral NSAIDs in the suggested order of pharmacological therapies.

6.7 What is the difference between topical capsaicin and topical NSAIDs?

Capsaicin has a unique action within the joint by interfering with pain transmission (see Q. 6.6). The clinical effect of topical NSAIDs is thought to be due to the anti-inflammatory effect of the NSAID within the joint and surrounding tissues. The advantage of a topical NSAID is that some drug level is achieved within the joint while avoiding the high serum levels seen with oral therapy.

6.8 Are rubefacients useful?

Rubefacients work by producing counter-irritation. This means that the irritation and erythema produced in the skin by these agents help to relieve pain in underlying muscles, tendons and joints. Many patients find the use of rubefacients provides comfort and subsequent reduction of pain. These products are safe and cheap and may be useful in mild OA.

PQ PATIENT QUESTIONS

6.9   Can I use topical creams I buy from my chemist as well as take my arthritis tablets?

This question should be addressed to your doctor or pharmacist as it is essential to know what medication you are taking.

The only topical cream that can be used regardless of which arthritis tablets you are taking is the modern equivalent of 'Fiery Jack' or 'horse liniment'. These products are called rubefacients and do not contain NSAIDs.

Pharmacological management 2: Analgesics

7

7.1   What is the role of simple analgesics in OA?

Simple analgesia (paracetamol/acetaminophen) is the mainstay of pharmaceutical management. It is the safest analgesic and should be taken, or at least tried, by all patients as their first choice of pain relief.

All analgesia is used to improve a patient's quality of life by relieving pain. This may be pain brought on by an everyday activity such as going shopping, hanging out washing, playing golf or bowls, or gardening.

For paracetamol to be most effective it is best to advise the patient to take the tablets before commencing an activity in order to prevent the pain building up so that it does not disrupt the patient's actions. Paracetamol can also be taken when the pain begins but it will then take 20 min before it has an effect.

Paracetamol may be used as an adjunct to other analgesia, especially in combination with codeine. Importantly, patients may take paracetamol as well as their NSAID (non-steroidal anti-inflammatory drug), thus improving the pain relief and even limiting the prescribed dose of NSAID.

Patients will need encouragement to take the paracetamol every 4 h, but this is essential to maintain ongoing pain relief.

7.2   When should compound analgesics be used?

Adding codeine to paracetamol produces analgesia greater than either drug used alone; in fact, there seems to be an additive effect. Evidence on single dosing for pain relief, after anaesthesia for tooth extraction, shows that paracetamol 600 mg + codeine 60 mg is equivalent to paracetamol 1 g. Research shows that the best combination is paracetamol 1 g + codeine 60 mg [number needed to treat (NNT) to give 50% pain relief=2] (*see Fig. 7.1*).

The message is that combining codeine with paracetamol is likely to give greater analgesia. In many patients, this is equivalent to taking fairly large doses of NSAIDs but with an almost negligible risk when paracetamol is used at therapeutic doses.

There is an expanding group of patients who should only take paracetamol or paracetamol–opioid combination. This group includes those patients who are asthmatic, have heart failure, have suffered a gastrointestinal bleed or perforation and are over 65 years of age.

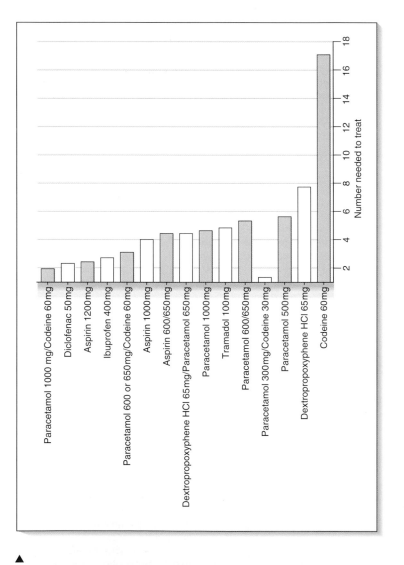

▲

Fig. 7.1 Pain analgesia ladder. From Moore RA, McQuay HJ 2000 Easy targets aren't always the right ones. Bandolier (http://www.jr2.ox.ac.uk/bandolier) with permission.

7.3   Are there any pro formas that give advice on the use of analgesia for pain relief?

The Oxford Pain Research website (*see Appendix 3*) has lots of information on it, including NNTs for the most common analgesics (NNT is the number of patients needing to be treated to give 50% pain relief). Remember that the patient is the one to respond to the drug or the dose chosen; the list and NNT also give an indication of the likelihood of failure.

The site also suggests a scheme (the 'three-pot' scheme) for treating patients with:

- Paracetamol alone
- Paracetamol plus codeine combined
- Ibuprofen/NSAIDs.

The 'pots' are used according to the amount of pain experienced and whether or not the patient can tolerate NSAIDs (*see Figs 7.2 and 7.3*). Importantly, the therapeutic dose of paracetamol must not be exceeded, so the repeat cycle for paracetamol must be noted.

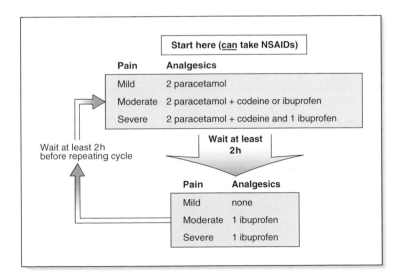

Fig. 7.2 The 'three-pot' scheme of analgesia for patients who can tolerate NSAIDs. From Moore RA, McQuay HJ 2000 Easy targets aren't always the right ones. Bandolier (http://www.jr2.ox.ac.uk/bandolier) with permission.

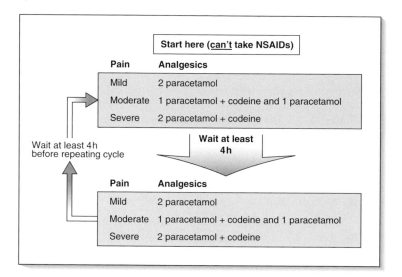

▲

Fig. 7.3 The 'three-pot' scheme of analgesia for patients who cannot tolerate NSAIDs. From Moore RA, McQuay HJ 2000 Easy targets aren't always the right ones. Bandolier (http://www.jr2.ox.ac.uk/bandolier) with permission.

7.4 What are the advantages of paracetamol?

- It is absolutely safe for all ages if taken according to the manufacturer's instructions.
- It does not cause serious perforations, ulcers or bleeds.
- It can be added to adequate doses of codeine (30 mg, 60 mg) to give excellent NNTs.
- It may be used to enhance a regimen using NSAIDs/COX-2 (cyclo-oxygenase-2) inhibitors.
- It does not have any cardiac toxicity and is thus safe for patients with cardiac disease.

7.5 What are the disadvantages of paracetamol?

The bitter taste does not help compliance. The main disadvantage is the half-life; regular 4-hourly dosing is required to keep up the therapeutic blood levels. The maximum dose of 4 g a day for an adult must not be exceeded. Patients must be warned to read all instructions on all medications that they are taking, especially any other analgesics (*see Q. 7.17*). Rarely do patients experience side-effects. Rashes and blood disorders are rare, as is acute pancreatitis after prolonged use.

7.6 Is liver failure a common side-effect from taking paracetamol?

 No. Paracetamol taken in therapeutic doses does not cause liver failure or cause renal damage. Remember, that a patient in liver failure, from whatever reason, can be given paracetamol for a headache or pain relief.

The literature shows that it is extremely rare for a person to exceed the therapeutic dose unintentionally. There is the potential for it to happen if the instructions are not read carefully, especially if the person is self-medicating. Patients who are taking prescribed medication and then self-prescribe with additional over-the-counter medications are at greatest risk of overdosing.

7.7 Does paracetamol relieve stiffness?

Paracetamol relieves pain but is not reputed to relieve stiffness in OA joints. Some patients report much more mobility when taking the drug on a regular basis.

7.8 Does paracetamol cause asthma?

No. Paracetamol can safely be given to asthmatics. It does not cause a wheeze or asthma in non-asthmatics.

7.9 There is a wide variation in the amount of codeine in compound analgesics. What is the correct dosage?

There is no set correct dose of codeine. The dosage appears to vary from one country to another. Britain tends to use smaller doses than many European countries. For instance, co-codamol contains 8 mg codeine + 500 mg paracetamol. Continental Europe standard would start at a dose of 30 mg; this fits much more with evidence from the pain analgesia ladder (*see Fig. 7.1*). Top of the ladder is paracetamol 1000 mg + codeine 60 mg. From this we can deduce that the preparation likely to help most people in severe pain is tablets containing codeine 30 mg + paracetamol 500 mg. The British National Formulary (BNF) lists a number of proprietary and non-proprietary preparations (co-codamol 30/500).

7.10 Is it better to use codeine phosphate alone or in combination with paracetamol?

The pain analgesia ladder (*see Fig. 7.1*) indicates that codeine alone is not as good as codeine plus paracetamol for severe pain; thus patients in severe pain require a combination of codeine + paracetamol. This can be given as a combination tablet (*see Q. 7.9*) or as individual tablets of paracetamol and codeine.

The 'three-pot' system (*see Figs 7.2 and 7.3*) advocates individual tablets so that patients can mix and match medication according to the severity of the pain and can adjust the dosage for specific activities or daily variations. For example, for moderate pain, paracetamol + codeine is recommended. The dose of codeine can be adjusted, and the pain analgesia ladder would suggest 30 mg or 60 mg rather than 8 mg.

7.11 What is the role of opiate drugs and their derivatives?

Codeine is used alone and in combination, usually with paracetamol. Adequate doses of codeine (30 mg, 60 mg) in combination with paracetamol are extremely effective and should be tried before resorting to other opiates or opiate derivatives.

Pethidine and morphine will rarely be required if patients are given good advice on managing their pain with codeine and paracetamol.

 Opiate derivatives promise a lot and can be useful in some individuals. However, finding which patients these are often causes frustration for doctors and patients alike as the NNTs are high and side-effects common.

7.12 Should aspirin be used to treat OA?

 There are multiple reasons and medical conditions for the use of aspirin but it is *not* recommended for OA as the doses needed for pain relief are likely to cause gastrointestinal side-effects.

Patients with OA and other medical conditions that require the use of aspirin should be on the lowest recommended dose. These patients are often elderly and are likely to be taking NSAIDs/COX-2 inhibitors. These factors place the individual at greater risk of gastrointestinal side-effects, which may be catastrophic. (*See also Ch. 8.*)

7.13 If the patient has had a perforation and doesn't respond to analgesics, what else may be prescribed?

 First, check which medication the patient has tried and when it is being taken. Is the dose of codeine adequate? (*See Q. 7.9.*) Has the patient tried other opiates or opiate derivatives? Perhaps the patient has tried all the alternatives and they have been inadequate or produced unacceptable side-effects. What else should be tried?

■ Topical treatments. The safest would be capsaicin cream, which reduces substance P in the nerve endings. This should certainly be tried on any joint amenable to topical treatment. It can also be used as an adjunct to analgesia (*see Q. 6.3*). Capsaicin is not an NSAID;

topical NSAIDs used correctly and not abused are an alternative to capsaicin.

■ Injections. These are definite alternatives to analgesics and should be tried for all joints, either in primary or secondary care. Steroid injections are certainly worthwhile, and in certain joints hyaluronan may be beneficial for some patients.

7.14 Should elderly patients only be given analgesics, or are NSAIDs or COX-2 inhibitors appropriate?

Any treatment given to a patient should be appropriate for the individual and their disease. Use the least potentially dangerous drugs as first choice (i.e. analgesics, including combination with adequate doses of codeine) to give pain relief that is acceptable to the patient.

Most patients can be managed this way, sometimes with the addition of topical treatments (e.g. capsaicin cream).

A few patients will require either the addition or the replacement of the analgesic with COX-2 (cyclo-oxygenase-2) inhibitors. The NICE guidelines give the advice that patients over 65 should be prescribed COX-2 inhibitors. The important principle is to strive to give patients maximum pain relief and mobility in the safest possible way whilst respecting the patient's views and opinions.

7.15 Do patients become intolerant of analgesics over time and require stronger or alternative drugs?

It is unlikely that patients will become intolerant of analgesics. Some of the reasons that patients may appear to be intolerant are listed in *Box 7.1*. Management will depend upon the likely cause of the 'intolerance'.

BOX 7.1 Reasons why patients may appear to be intolerant to analgesics

■ OA may have progressed or there is an additional complication such as the femoral head may have collapsed

■ The patient may not be taking the analgesics as prescribed

■ The patient may be depressed and so the pain threshold will have changed

■ Exclude 'red flags' (infection, trauma/fracture, cancer)

7.16   What is the purpose of taking medication?

Most medications for arthritis are given to relieve pain. It is the pain that makes life difficult for patients. Relieving pain may also relieve joint stiffness, allow a better night's sleep, allow a person to engage in more activities and generally make life more pleasant.

It is not essential to take tablets for arthritis but they are one form of medication used to try to relieve pain and other symptoms. It is possible to use injections and topical creams and gels. A non-medication form of treatment is physiotherapy; heat and cold may also be used. Complementary practitioners may offer other forms of therapy such as reflexology, homeopathy and aromatherapy. All of the modalities may be used alone or in combination.

7.17   Is it more dangerous to take eight paracetamol a day than one NSAID?

No. Paracetamol is absolutely safe if taken according to the manufacturer's instructions.

The risk of dying from gastrointestinal problems after at least 2 months on an NSAID is of the order of 1 in 1200. This is a finite risk. The risk of dying of therapeutic doses of paracetamol alone or in combination with codeine is negligible.

7.18   Paracetamol medication carries a warning about liver disease: is it safe?

Yes, paracetamol is safe, but it is important not to exceed the stated maximum dose. Always read and follow the instructions that are written on the box and on the leaflet included in the package. Importantly, paracetamol is not contraindicated for patients who are pregnant or have asthma. It is safe for people of all ages, including children, as long as the instructions are followed. It can be given to patients with liver disease for headaches.

7.19   I am going on holiday abroad; can I buy my analgesics in other countries?

You would be well advised to take an adequate supply of medication with you. This is because there are many different formulations of very similar products around the world and it is not always easy to obtain an exact match. For example, the amount of paracetamol in a tablet can be 325 mg, 500 mg or 625 mg, and now there are also slow-release tablets in some countries. If you do need to buy tablets abroad, you will need advice from the local pharmacist and you will have to supply as many details as possible about your medication.

Pharmacological management 3: NSAIDs and COX-2 inhibitors

8

PQ PATIENT QUESTIONS

NON-STEROIDAL ANTI-INFLAMMATORY DRUGS (NSAIDS)

8.1 What are the benefits of NSAIDs over simple and compound analgesics?

NSAIDs (non-steroidal anti-inflammatory drugs) have anti-inflammatory effects as well as analgesic effects. These anti-inflammatory effects are useful in treating conditions in which inflammation is present (e.g. inflammatory arthritis and gout). It is often stated that because OA is not an inflammatory condition it is not justifiable to prescribe a NSAID to patients with OA. However, it is thought that there is a degree of inflammation present in joints affected by OA, both in the development stages and especially at times of flare. Conventional inflammatory markers do not show an inflammatory response at these times, but it may be that sensitive markers for this type of inflammation have not yet been developed. From a clinical point of view, some patients seem to gain a significant benefit from NSAID therapy over that of simple and compound analgesics.

NSAIDs can have serious side-effects, particularly on the gastrointestinal system by causing peptic ulceration, perforations and bleeding (PUBs); they may also cause renal problems and aggravate heart failure by causing fluid retention.

NSAIDs should only be prescribed where there is a clear reason and where benefits would outweigh the risks. On the other hand, analgesics themselves often have significant side-effects, particularly in elderly patients, causing constipation, headache, dizziness and confusion. The problems of pain and disability need to be addressed together with side-effects of therapy as all of these factors affect an individual's quality of life. Each patient requires an individual assessment of his or her own circumstances, looking at these issues and providing the patient with sufficient information to allow informed choices to be made. Despite knowing the risks of NSAID therapy, many patients would prefer to take an anti-inflammatory drug because of the improved symptom control and ease of administration. The dosage regimens for NSAIDs, usually once or twice daily, are often much simpler than those for analgesics and patients often prefer them for this reason.

There seems to be an individual reaction to NSAID therapy and some patients derive considerable benefit with relief of pain and stiffness while others do equally well with analgesic therapy. Around 60% will respond to any NSAID whereas others may respond only to certain NSAIDs. If one drug is not effective when prescribed at a reasonable dose and for up to 3 weeks, then it is worth trying another to assess its efficacy.

8.2 When should NSAIDs be used?

Provided there are no contraindications (*see Qs 8.6, 8.8 and 8.9*), NSAID therapy should be considered in patients with the following conditions:

■ Inflammatory arthritis
■ Gout
■ Osteoarthritis (following failure of analgesic therapy or for inflammatory flares)
■ Back pain.

8.3 What are the 'rules' for using NSAIDs?

As a general principle, NSAIDs should be prescribed initially at the lowest recommended dose and only one NSAID should be prescribed at any one time. It is important to ask the patient whether they are taking anything from the pharmacy as they may be taking over-the-counter ibuprofen without realizing that it is an NSAID.

NSAIDs should only be prescribed where there is an obvious clinical need and where there are no contraindications (*see Q. 8.4*).

8.4 How does the NICE guidance affect the prescribing of NSAIDs?

The NICE guidance suggests that standard NSAIDs should be used in preference to COX-2 (cyclo-oxygenase-2) inhibitors in all patients unless they fall into certain high-risk groups (*see Box 8.1*).

NICE also emphasizes that NSAIDs should only be prescribed if there is an obvious clinical need, that long-term use should be avoided if possible and that patients taking NSAIDs should be monitored to ascertain the continuing need for long-term treatment.

NICE has also recommended that standard NSAIDs, together with gastric protection if required, are used in patients with cardiovascular disease and those on long-term low-dose aspirin even if they fall into the categories for the use of COX-2 inhibitors.

BOX 8.1 High-risk groups contraindicating prescribing of NSAIDs

■ Those aged over 65
■ Those with a past or present history of peptic ulceration
■ Those taking other medications known to increase the risk of gastrointestinal problems
■ Those who require long-term use of NSAIDs at high dose
■ Those with other serious concomitant disease

BOX 8.2 Adverse effects of NSAIDs

- Gastrointestinal effects: nausea, diarrhoea, abdominal pain, ulceration, bleeding, perforation
- Hypersensitivity reactions: rashes, angioedema, bronchospasm
- Central nervous system effects: headache, dizziness, insomnia
- Blood dyscrasias
- Renal problems
- Fluid retention: may precipitate heart failure, especially in the elderly

8.5   What are the main side-effects of NSAIDs?

NSAIDs can have adverse effects on several systems of the body (*see Box 8.2*).

8.6   What are the main drug interactions with NSAIDs?

There are many potential interactions of NSAIDs with other commonly prescribed drugs (*see Box 8.3*). Some interactions are specific for one particular NSAID; others apply to all NSAIDs—i.e. a 'class effect'. For a full list of interactions see the British National Formulary (BNF).

8.7   What are the main limitations to the use of NSAIDs?

NSAIDs are symptom-relievers rather than cures for inflammatory and painful conditions. They are useful in patients with inflammatory arthritis such as rheumatoid arthritis (RA) during the development of

BOX 8.3 The most important drug interactions of NSAIDs/ COX-2 inhibitors

- Angiotensin-converting enzyme (ACE) inhibitors and angiotensin-II antagonists
- Other oral NSAIDs
- Quinolone antibiotics
- Anticoagulants
- Sulphonylureas
- Phenytoin
- Antivirals
- Ciclosporin and tacrolimus
- Methotrexate
- Diuretics
- Lithium
- Probenecid

the condition, and for inflammatory flares. Ideally, when disease-modifying anti-rheumatic drugs (DMARDs) begin to exert their effect in inflammatory arthritis, the dose of NSAID can be reduced and possibly totally discontinued. The toxicity of NSAIDs has been shown by Fries et al (1990) to be similar or even worse than that of DMARDs; thus one of the aims of good long-term treatment of RA with DMARDs is to reduce the patient's exposure to NSAIDs. Despite good DMARD control, however, there are many patients who find it impossible to discontinue their NSAID because of the relief of pain and stiffness they experience while using these drugs.

8.8 What are the main contraindications for the use of NSAIDs?

The main contraindications and cautions for NSAIDs are:

- A history of hypersensitivity to aspirin or other NSAIDs
- Pregnancy and breastfeeding
- Coagulation defects
- Active peptic ulceration.

8.9 What are the relative contraindications for the use of NSAIDs?

Relative contraindications for NSAIDs are:

- History of gastrointestinal bleeding or ulceration
- Renal, cardiac or hepatic impairment
- Asthma
- Relevant concomitant medication (*see* Q. 8.6).

8.10 Which NSAID should be prescribed?

Normally ibuprofen is the first NSAID that should be prescribed. It is thought that ibuprofen is the least likely NSAID to cause gastrointestinal problems, but this may be the result of doctors using low doses of the drug. In fact, many patients find that the commonly prescribed dose of 400—600 mg three times daily is relatively ineffective. If the dose of ibuprofen is increased, the side-effect profile changes to reflect this and the number of gastrointestinal side-effects increases.

Other NSAIDs commonly prescribed in the UK are diclofenac, naproxen and nabumetone. Meloxicam and etodolac are now regarded as selective COX-2 inhibitors rather than standard NSAIDs.

8.11 When should ibuprofen not be prescribed as the first choice?

Ibuprofen at standard doses is perceived as a 'weak' NSAID. If strong anti-inflammatory and analgesic control is required then it may be sensible to prescribe another NSAID as first choice. It is also important to ask the patient what drugs they have been taking 'over the counter'. You may find that many will have tried a variety of analgesics and also ibuprofen at different doses before coming to a consultation.

8.12 How soon do NSAIDs/COX-2 inhibitors work?

NSAIDs/COX-2 inhibitors have two forms of action: analgesic and anti-inflammatory. Most NSAIDs/COX-2 inhibitors will show an analgesic effect after 1 week, but an anti-inflammatory response may take up to 3 weeks. If there is no response after this time, then another NSAID should be tried.

8.13 Is it true that NSAIDs/COX-2 inhibitors help with patients' stiffness from their OA?

Patients certainly find that NSAIDs and COX-2 inhibitors help the stiffness associated with arthritis. This is more apparent in rheumatoid arthritis (RA) than in OA as the stiffness of RA tends to be longer-lasting. Many patients with OA find that their stiffness only lasts a short time after a period of immobility. For others, stiffness can last for up to 30 min and becomes a real problem; the use of an NSAID or COX-2 inhibitor for these patients is often very beneficial.

8.14 Is there any contraindication for the use of NSAIDs/COX-2 inhibitors if a patient is already taking an ACE inhibitor?

NSAIDs may interact with ACE (angiotensin-converting enzyme) inhibitors and angiotensin-II antagonists, reducing the hypotensive effect and increasing the risk of renal impairment and hyperkalaemia.

8.15 How common are central nervous system side-effects in patients taking NSAIDs/COX-2 inhibitors?

All side-effects are too common if you are the patient with a problem from a side-effect, but they are not common enough to warn every patient about them. These drugs do cross the blood–brain barrier (note their use in headaches and migraine) and a few patients will have side-effects ranging widely from headaches, drowsiness, dizziness and vertigo to apprehension and depression. These are all distressing but apprehension and depression, when they occur, may be very debilitating. These side-effects may upset the doctor–patient relationship if the patient has not been warned about them.

8.16 How common are renal problems with NSAIDs/COX-2 inhibitors?

In patients with already compromised renal function, the use of NSAIDs/COX-2 inhibitors may provoke renal failure. If an NSAID is clinically essential for such a patient, the dose should be kept as low as possible and renal function should be monitored. NSAID/COX-2 inhibitors can rarely cause papillary necrosis or interstitial fibrosis and this may lead to renal failure.

8.17 When is it important to check urea and electrolytes for patients who have been prescribed NSAIDs?

If the patient is known to have a degree of renal failure and it is essential that he or she is given NSAID therapy, then it is important to review renal function at regular intervals. Elderly patients often have age-related compromised renal function and, again, if an NSAID is really required then renal function should be checked at regular intervals, although there are no specific recommendations for this.

NSAIDs interact with ACE inhibitors and they should probably not be prescribed together unless essential. If co-prescription is required, then renal function, including electrolytes, should ideally be monitored.

8.18 How often should liver function tests be undertaken for patients taking diclofenac?

There are no specific recommendations for the monitoring of liver function in patients taking diclofenac and there is no mention of this on the product data sheet. If a patient is known to have compromised hepatic function, it would be sensible to avoid NSAIDs in general, but if it is essential to prescribe an NSAID then diclofenac should be avoided. If a patient is having short-term therapy with diclofenac, then monitoring of LFTs is probably not required. If, however, a patient requires long-term therapy, then checking LFTs after 2–3 months of taking the drug and again at intervals thereafter is probably sensible.

8.19 If a patient is taking a diuretic for blood pressure problems can NSAIDs still be prescribed?

The use of a diuretic for blood pressure control is not a contraindication to the use of an NSAID. However, there is the possibility that there may be some interaction between the two drugs, and there may be some loss of blood pressure control. These patients will therefore require closer monitoring of blood pressure and possibly the addition of other therapy to maintain good control, especially if it is anticipated that the NSAID will be required therapy in the longer term.

8.20 If a patient is taking aspirin for heart problems can NSAIDs still be prescribed and, if so, which NSAIDs are preferable?

Current recommendations suggest that two NSAIDs should not be prescribed together. It has been shown that even low-dose aspirin alone can cause gastrointestinal bleeds (*see Q. 8.27*). There is, however, an increasing number of patients on low-dose aspirin (75 mg daily) for cardiovascular or cerebrovascular prophylaxis and many other patients buy low-dose aspirin over the counter because they have heard it may be of benefit. It has been thought that prescription of an NSAID, if clinically necessary, to a patient on low-dose aspirin has a slight added risk, provided there are no specific gastrointestinal risk factors, but is probably reasonably safe. However, a recently reported study from the University of Dundee Medicine Monitoring Unit has shown that patients with cardiovascular disease who were on aspirin and who took ibuprofen were almost twice as likely to die within the study period as those on aspirin alone, allowing for other risk factors. Results also showed that other NSAIDs were not associated with an increased risk of death, suggesting that aspirin and ibuprofen may have some interaction potential. This is an important finding, especially as we are encouraged to prescribe ibuprofen as our first-choice NSAID. Patients also have access to ibuprofen over the counter as well as to aspirin and may well be taking both without the knowledge of their medical advisor.

8.21 Do NSAIDs/COX-2 inhibitors have an effect on blood sugar levels?

There is no evidence that NSAIDs interfere with blood sugar levels or diabetic control.

8.22 Do all NSAIDs carry the same risk of perforation/ulceration/ bleeding (PUBs)?

The Committee for the Safety of Medicines (CSM) in 1994 looked at the relative safety of seven NSAIDs with regard to serious upper gastrointestinal events (*see Box 8.4*). They found that ibuprofen had the lowest risk, diclofenac, naproxen, ketoprofen and piroxicam intermediate risk (with piroxicam at the higher end of the intermediate group) and azapropazone the highest risk (*see Box 8.5*). It should be remembered that this list does not include the newer drugs such as meloxicam, etodolac, nabumetone, rofecoxib, celecoxib and etoricoxib.

8.23 How does the dose of NSAIDs affect gastric side-effects?

There does seem to be a relationship between increase in gastric side-effects and increasing dose of NSAID. To limit exposure it is suggested that the lowest effective dose should be given for the shortest effective time. Ibuprofen is usually suggested as the first choice in NSAID therapy because it is least likely to produce serious gastrointestinal problems. It is also perceived by patients and doctors as a weaker NSAID; in other words, less effective in terms of symptom control. If the dose of ibuprofen is increased

> **BOX 8.4 CSM advice on the relative safety of seven NSAIDs**
>
> **CSM advice (gastrointestinal side-effects)**
> Evidence on the relative safety of seven non-selective NSAIDs indicates differences in the risks of serious upper gastrointestinal side-effects. Azapropazone is associated with the highest risk and ibuprofen with the lowest; piroxicam, ketoprofen, indometacin, naproxen and diclofenac are associated with intermediate risks (possibly higher in the case of piroxicam). Selective inhibitors of cyclo-oxygenase-2 are associated with a lower risk of serious upper gastrointestinal side-effects than non-selective NSAIDs.
>
> Recommendations are that NSAIDs associated with low risk (e.g. ibuprofen) are generally preferred, to start at the lowest recommended dose, not to use more than one oral NSAID at a time, and to remember that all NSAIDs (including selective inhibitors of cyclo-oxygenase-2) are contraindicated in patients with peptic ulceration. The CSM also contraindicates non-selective NSAIDs in patients with a history of peptic ulceration.
>
> The combination of an NSAID and low-dose aspirin may increase the risk of gastrointestinal side-effects; this combination should only be used if absolutely necessary and the patient monitored closely.
>
> **CSM warning (asthma)**
> Any degree of worsening of asthma may be related to the ingestion of NSAIDs, either prescribed or (in the case of ibuprofen and others) purchased over the counter.
>
> Source: BNF 44.

> **BOX 8.5 Restrictions on the use of azapropazone**
>
> ■ Only in rheumatoid arthritis (RA), ankylosing spondylitis and acute gout if other NSAIDs have been tried and failed
> ■ Maximum daily dose of 600 mg for RA and ankylosing spondylitis in patients aged over 60
> ■ Totally contraindicated in patients with a history of peptic ulceration

to give potentially better symptom control, it has been shown that the incidence of gastric side-effects also rises, comparable with other NSAIDs.

8.24 Do enteric-coated preparations of NSAIDs reduce gastrointestinal problems?

The main reason for the development of PUBs associated with an NSAID is thought to be related to the circulating levels of the drug. This would not be affected by using an enteric-coated preparation. Dyspeptic symptoms, however, may be reduced by an enteric coating.

8.25 Do slow-release preparations, suppositories and injection preparations cause as many serious side-effects as oral preparations?

The mechanism of damage to the gastric mucosa (PUBs) by NSAIDs is thought to be due to a combination of local effects of the drug on the stomach lining and systemic effects of the circulating drug. For this reason, the manner of giving the drug is less important than the levels attained. Absorption may be less with some other methods of administering the drug than with oral preparations and this may mean lower drug levels and therefore fewer gastrointestinal side-effects.

8.26 Should slow-release preparations be used to minimize local stomach intolerance?

The stomach problems associated with NSAIDs are thought to be the result of both systemic effects due to the levels of circulating drug and local effects due to the direct contact of the NSAID with the gastric mucosa. Slow-release preparations may slightly reduce the time of local exposure of the gastric mucosa to the irritant drug, but there is little evidence that this reduces gastric side-effects. Other advantages of slow-release preparations, which have a longer half-life, are that they provide a simpler dosing schedule and a more even level of drug in the body by avoiding peaks and troughs.

8.27 What happens to the risk of gastrointestinal PUBs when aspirin is combined with NSAIDs?

The risk of PUBs (perforation, ulceration, bleeding) increases when aspirin is given together with an NSAID. Many patients are taking low-dose aspirin on a daily basis as prophylaxis or secondary prevention for cardiovascular and cerebrovascular problems and the co-prescribing of aspirin with NSAID is a very common occurrence. It is thought by some that using enteric-coated aspirin can reduce the risk by reducing local irritation to the gastric mucosa. Many others feel, however, that this is not useful as the main risk for the development of gastrointestinal problems relates to the level of drug in the body tissues and not to local factors acting directly on the gastric mucosa. Many of the patients taking aspirin prophylaxis will be in the older age groups and many will have cardiovascular disease for which COX-2 inhibitors are relatively contraindicated. If it is thought necessary to co-prescribe aspirin together with an NSAID, then the best combination for these patients would be using an NSAID together with a proton pump inhibitor as gastric protection. (Remember that H_2-receptor blockers only help the indigestion, and do not have any effect on the incidence of PUBs.)

8.28 Should co-prescription of an NSAID with some form of gastric protection always be used?

Younger patients and those with no obvious risk factors should not routinely be prescribed gastric protection with NSAID. However, all patients should be warned of the possibility of gastrointestinal problems developing. The presence of dyspepsia does not necessarily mean that serious problems are developing; in fact, the majority of patients presenting with major gastrointestinal events have no history of dyspepsia. It is therefore impossible to predict accurately who is going to sustain a serious gastrointestinal event, but if patients within the high-risk categories are treated with COX-2 inhibitors or NSAIDs with gastric protection then this will go a long way to reducing the number of PUBs. In an ideal world, everyone taking an NSAID would be given some form of gastric protection, but this would certainly not be cost-effective. It is also worth remembering that some of the drugs used for gastric protection can cause side-effects themselves. Misoprostol is often poorly tolerated because of abdominal pain and diarrhoea, and proton pump inhibitors (PPIs) can also cause diarrhoea.

NSAIDs should not be used in certain clinical situations or in those taking certain concomitant medications (*see Qs 8.6, 8.8 and 8.9*).

A long-term study by MacDonald et al in Tayside in 1997 showed that the risk of NSAIDs was constant during continuous therapy and also that there was an excess risk carried over after the end of the exposure for at least a year.

8.29 Has yellow card reporting confirmed the relative gastrointestinal safety of NSAIDs?

The yellow card reporting system has certainly not confirmed the relative gastrointestinal safety of NSAIDs. In fact, it has had the opposite result and has pinpointed the fact that there are serious problems with the gastric safety of NSAIDs. This is very important because, although each individual GP will probably only see one serious gastrointestinal event caused by an NSAID every few years, the actual numbers throughout the country are certainly significant. It has been reported that there are around 2000 deaths each year attributable to the use of NSAIDs. Another way of stating the risk is that 1 in 1200 patients who have taken NSAIDs for at least 2 months will die from gastrointestinal complications (Tramer et al 2000).

8.30 What evidence is there to suggest that an NSAID prescription should be reviewed?

A study performed in Bristol by Dieppe et al (1993) enrolled patients who had been taking regular NSAID therapy for OA knee. Half of the number were randomized to placebo and half to diclofenac in a double-blind controlled trial. Some of the patients who had previously been established on an NSAID remained well-controlled on placebo over a 2-year period with paracetamol as escape therapy, suggesting that they had not really required the NSAID for symptom relief. On the other hand, some who had previously been established on NSAID and who were now given placebo suffered a significant flare of symptoms, some even requiring withdrawal from the study. These patients obviously required NSAID for symptom relief. It is therefore probably sensible to review the need for long-term NSAID therapy to avoid inappropriate usage and the subsequent increased likelihood of side-effects. Patients who are hypertensive may lose control of hypertension on NSAID therapy and this will need monitoring. Patients who have controlled or incipient heart failure and are given an NSAID may develop increased fluid retention which may be sufficient to precipitate frank symptoms; again, if such patients really require NSAID therapy, they should be reviewed regularly. Similarly, patients with renal or hepatic impairment should be monitored and reviewed at regular intervals.

Some patients may be started on NSAID therapy for a short-term indication and may continue to request this as a repeat prescription without any review taking place. In these days of computerized repeat prescription systems, it is possible for such a prescription to be repeated without doctor or pharmacist review. Most repeat prescribing systems can be amended to highlight the need for review at certain designated intervals and it would be sensible for this to be incorporated by agreement within the practice of a suitable time interval.

8.31 Should patients be tested for *Helicobacter pylori* before being given long-term NSAIDs?

A recent study (Labenz et al 2002) has shown that eradicating *H. pylori* before commencing a 5-week course of diclofenac reduced the rate of peptic ulceration almost to zero. In patients who were *H. pylori* positive and who had eradication, the incidence of peptic ulceration was 1%, whereas in those who were *H. pylori* positive but who were left untreated the peptic ulceration rate was 6%. These findings would suggest that we should be testing for *H. pylori* before commencing long-term treatment with NSAIDs and, if positive, giving eradication treatment.

8.32 What is the suggested pathway for the pharmacological management of OA?

The Primary Care Rheumatology Society Guidelines for the management of knee OA suggest that the order of drug treatment should be:

■ Paracetamol
■ Topical NSAIDs/capsaicin
■ Compound analgesics
■ Oral NSAIDs
■ Steroid injection
■ Intra-articular hyaluronan injection.

The American College of Rheumatology Guidelines (Hochberg et al 1995) suggest a very similar hierarchy, although they suggest that if there is an effusion or local signs of inflammation then steroid injection should be used sooner.

CYCLO-OXYGENASE-2 (COX-2) INHIBITORS

8.33 What is a simple explanation of COX?

Anti-inflammatory drugs are thought to work by interfering with the production of prostaglandins from their precursor, arachidonic acid, by inhibiting the enzyme cyclo-oxygenase (COX). Prostaglandins are responsible not only for mediating inflammation and pain but also for protecting the gastric mucosa, renal function and platelet activity. When a drug such as an NSAID inhibits prostaglandin production, this results in the reduction of inflammation and pain—a desired effect—while at the same time reducing protection to gastric mucosa, renal and platelet function—undesired effects. An ideal anti-inflammatory, therefore, would be one that preserved the protective effects of prostaglandins on stomach, kidneys and platelets while at the same time blocked pain and inflammation.

It was discovered in 1991 that there are two isoforms of COX known as COX-1 and COX-2. COX-1 is known as the constitutive (or housekeeping) form and is responsible for the production of those prostaglandins that are required for the maintenance of normal endocrine and renal function, haemostasis and the protection of gastric mucosa. COX-2 is known as the inducible (or inflammatory) form and is responsible for the production of those prostaglandins that lead to inflammation and subsequent pain.

COX-2 inhibitors are thought to act by selectively blocking COX-2, thereby reducing pain and inflammation, but not blocking COX-1, thereby preserving the protective effects of prostaglandins on the stomach, kidneys and platelets. Standard NSAIDs are thought to block both COX-1 and COX-2, reducing inflammation but at the same time blocking the protective role of COX-1 and producing adverse effects, particularly to the gastric mucosa (*see Fig. 8.1*).

8.34 When talking about COX, what is inducible COX-2?

Arachidonic acid, which is formed from membrane phospholipids, produces prostaglandins by means of the enzyme cyclo-oxygenase (COX). This enzyme has been shown to have two isoforms: cyclo-oxygenase-1 (COX-1) and cyclo-oxygenase-2 (COX-2). COX-2 is responsible for the

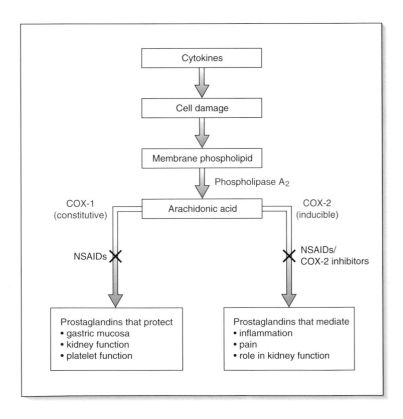

▲

Fig. 8.1 Simplified version of part of the inflammatory cascade showing sites of action of NSAIDs and COX-2 inhibitors.

production of those prostaglandins that lead to inflammation and is known as the inducible (or inflammatory) form of the enzyme.

8.35   When talking about COX, what is constitutive COX-1?

Arachidonic acid, which is formed from membrane phospholipids, produces prostaglandins by means of the enzyme cyclo-oxygenase (COX). This enzyme has been shown to have two isoforms: cyclo-oxygenase-1 (COX-1) and cyclo-oxygenase-2 (COX-2). COX-1 is responsible for the production of those prostaglandins that protect gastric mucosa, renal function and platelet activity and is known as the constitutive or housekeeping enzyme (*see Q. 8.2*).

8.36   What are the contraindications for the use of COX-2 inhibitors?

The contraindications to the use of COX-2 inhibitors are similar to those of NSAIDs in general (*see Qs 8.8 and 8.9*).

8.37   What are the relative contraindications for the use of COX-2 inhibitors?

Again, these are similar to those of NSAIDs (*see Qs 8.8, 8.9 and 8.14*). The CSM (Committee for the Safety of Medicines) has placed specific advice regarding rofecoxib; namely, that it should not be prescribed to patients with severe congestive cardiac failure and that caution should be exercised in patients with a history of cardiac failure, left ventricular failure or hypertension and in patients with oedema for any other reason. Reviewing FDA (US Food and Drug Administration) data would suggest this advice should be applied to celecoxib also (i.e. be careful in these patients when using NSAIDs or COX-2 inhibitors).

8.38   What is the main reason for prescribing a COX-2 inhibitor?

The main reason for prescribing a COX-2 inhibitor is to protect the gastrointestinal tract from the development of perforations, ulceration and bleeding (PUBs) (Bombardier et al 2000, Silverstein et al 2000). These complications are more common in the elderly, those with a past history of peptic ulceration and those with serious co-morbidities or taking other drugs that increase the risk of gastrointestinal bleeding.

8.39   What are the rules for using COX-2 inhibitors?

NICE guidance (National Institute for Clinical Excellence 2001) suggests that those at highest risk for developing PUBs include those patients aged over 65, those with a past history of peptic ulceration and those taking co-prescriptions of other drugs such as steroid therapy which may increase the risk of a gastrointestinal bleed. Other high-risk groups include those with serious co-morbidities and those who require long-term use of anti-inflammatory therapy.

If patients in any of these groups require anti-inflammatory treatment, the use of a COX-2 inhibitor rather than an NSAID is recommended. These rules, however, should not be prescriptive and, as in many things in medicine, clinical judgement is the most important factor.

There is some controversy over the use of COX-2 inhibitors in patients with coronary artery disease and in those taking low-dose aspirin. It is thought that COX-2 inhibitors may have an adverse effect on cardiovascular disease. Also, as many patients with cardiovascular disease take daily low-dose aspirin, which can increase the risk of PUBs, the benefit of using a COX-2 inhibitor to decrease gastrointestinal adverse events is reduced in these patients. In this instance, the use of a standard NSAID together with a proton pump inhibitor (PPI) is probably the best option. Remember that the PPI will only reduce the risk by about half.

8.40   If giving a COX-2 inhibitor reduces the risk of PUBs by 50%, does co-prescribing a PPI reduce this risk further?

At present there is no evidence that co-prescribing a PPI (proton pump inhibitor) further reduces the risk of a gastrointestinal bleed.

8.41   Are there any patients that should be given a COX-2 inhibitor and a PPI/misoprostol?

Although there is no evidence that a PPI further reduces the risk of a gastrointestinal bleed, there may be some patients who have a medical history that puts them into a very high-risk group and in whom the prescription of an anti-inflammatory is essential for clinical reasons. In these cases, which are probably relatively few in number, it may be necessary to provide further gastric protection by co-prescribing a PPI together with a COX-2 inhibitor.

8.42   If a patient suffers from indigestion when taking a COX-2 inhibitor, what should be done?

Indigestion is a side-effect of both NSAIDs and COX-2 inhibitors. The development of dyspepsia is not necessarily a sign that the patient is developing peptic ulceration, as often the most serious

> gastrointestinal side-effects caused by anti-inflammatories are initially asymptomatic. If the COX-2 inhibitor can be stopped in a patient with dyspepsia, this is certainly the best solution. If the drug must be continued on clinical grounds, then the addition of an H_2-receptor blocker may resolve the symptoms. If not, it may be worth trying a different COX-2 inhibitor or a NSAID together with a PPI.

8.43 Should patients at risk of PUBs be referred for a gastroscopy before starting taking a COX-2 inhibitor?

There is no evidence that such a strategy would prevent the development of PUBs once the patient had started therapy. From the endoscopy studies that have been performed on patients on NSAIDs and COX-2 inhibitors, it has been found that many patients develop peptic ulceration in the first few weeks of therapy. The mucosa then seems to develop some resistance and these asymptomatic ulcers heal without causing any clinical problems. It may therefore be that the timing of the endoscopy is very important in relation to interpretation of any findings.

From an economic point of view, gastroscopy prior to therapy would almost certainly not be cost-effective.

8.44 If COX-2 inhibitors rarely cause serious gastrointestinal side-effects, do they help the healing of ulcers?

There is no evidence that COX-2 inhibitors help ulcers to heal. They are thought to have a neutral effect on gastric mucosa rather than an actual healing effect.

8.45 What are the differences between the recently launched COX-2 inhibitors and meloxicam and etodolac?

Rofecoxib, celecoxib and etoricoxib are thought to inhibit cyclo-oxygenase-2 (COX-2), the inducible isoform of COX, whereas meloxicam and etodolac are thought to have high COX-2 selectivity rather than complete inhibition.

8.46 Does a patient have to stop taking NSAIDs/COX-2 inhibitors if they are to be given a steroid injection?

There is no reason why patients should have to stop treatment with NSAID/COX-2 inhibitor because they are having a steroid injection. Some patients are treated with steroid injections because they have contraindications to the use of anti-inflammatory drugs, but for most patients with no specific contraindications it is sensible to continue analgesic or NSAID/COX-2 inhibitor therapy.

8.47 **The 'nuisance' side-effect profile of drugs causes some patients to stop taking the medication. Is there a difference in this profile between standard NSAIDs and COX-2 inhibitors?**

The main 'nuisance' side-effects of anti-inflammatory drugs are dyspepsia, fluid retention, loss of hypertension control and reduction of renal function. These side-effects appear to be similar with both standard NSAIDs and COX-2 inhibitors.

8.48 **Are the first-generation COX-2 inhibitors more powerful at relieving pain?**

COX-2 inhibitors seem to have a similar profile to NSAIDs in terms of their efficacy as pain-relieving anti-inflammatory drugs. High-dose rofecoxib at a dose of 25–50 mg now has a licence for short-term acute pain relief in postoperative pain and dysmenorrhoea. Importantly, the side-effect profile does not appear to have changed with this dose increase. This is in contradistinction to the use of higher doses of a standard NSAID.

8.49 **What further advances in COX-2 inhibition technology can be expected?**

We are already seeing more potent inhibitors of COX-2 brought to the market (e.g. etoricoxib). It is difficult to predict what other advances are likely. Obviously new side-chains are a possibility or attaching similar compounds, such as nitric oxide (naproxen NO, which is still under research, is one example using a standard NSAID). Any advance to help arthritic patients will be welcome.

8.50 **Has the yellow card reporting confirmed the relative safety of COX-2 inhibitors?**

The Medical Control Agency's Pharmacovigilance Group has analysed the yellow card reports for ten years (1990–2000) for two COX-2 inhibitors (rofecoxib and celecoxib) and for standard NSAIDs (diclofenac, naproxen and ibuprofen). The results show a higher rate of adverse gastrointestinal events for the two COX-2 inhibitors compared with the standard NSAIDs. It is difficult to know whether this is a true reflection of the problem for two main reasons:

- As COX-2 inhibitors are perceived to be safe for the stomach, patients with a history of PUBs (perforation, ulceration, bleeding) who might not previously have been prescribed an NSAID are now being treated with a COX-2 inhibitor.
- As COX-2 inhibitors are relatively new drugs, adverse events are more likely to be reported, whereas a gastrointestinal event with a standard

NSAID may not be reported on a yellow card as those side-effects are already well known.

Another study from Northern Ireland has reported that nearly 16 000 patients who had not been prescribed a standard NSAID previously because they were at high risk of a gastrointestinal event had subsequently been prescribed a COX-2 inhibitor.

The improved gastrointestinal safety profile seen with COX-2 inhibitors may be reduced if these drugs are prescribed solely to high-risk patients.

PQ PATIENT QUESTIONS

8.51   I have read that NSAIDs interfere with my blood pressure tablets, is this true?

Yes, it is true. NSAIDs tend to make people retain water and this tendency and other properties of NSAIDs may cause a slight rise in patients' blood pressure. This rise may be significant in some patients if blood pressure control is not ideal. NSAIDs should not be given to patients on ACE (angiotensin-converting enzyme) inhibitors unless a careful watch is kept on renal function and potassium levels.

8.52   Can I buy ibuprofen (Nurofen) from my chemist to take on my bad days as well as the tablets I get from my doctor?

No. It has been shown to be dangerous to mix more than one NSAID and ibuprofen (Nurofen) because ibuprofen (Nurofen) is an NSAID and it is likely that the arthritis tablets that you are taking will be a type of NSAID. Please discuss this subject with your pharmacist or doctor and so avoid the risks of serious stomach problems.

8.53   My doctor has given me some tablets for my arthritis but warned me that they might cause indigestion or serious stomach problems. I have got severe pain in my joints but I am really worried about taking these tablets. Can you advise?

Many tablets cause indigestion and NSAIDs may cause stomach bleeding and other stomach problems. Doctors try to limit these risks by not prescribing certain drugs to patients who have had serious stomach problems in the past. Pharmaceutical companies have developed new NSAIDs called COX-2 inhibitors which have been shown to lessen these risks, but these drugs do not eliminate all the problems/risks. The National Institute of Clinical Excellence (NICE) has stated that COX-2 inhibitors rather than the 'older' NSAIDs should be prescribed to patients over 65.

Unfortunately, some patients may still develop stomach problems and nowadays doctors have an obligation to warn patients about them.

8.54 Will the medication do more than help the pain?

The usual reason to give arthritis medication is to help relieve pain, but NSAIDs will also decrease stiffness and so improve your mobility.

8.55 Will I have to take/use the medication every day?

Most medication for arthritis is given to relieve pain and stiffness and so improve mobility and generally make life more pleasant. Some people will find that they do not need to take tablets all the time; if they are lucky they may only need to take them on the bad days or on the days they are more active. Other people will have to take medication for arthritis on a regular daily basis.

8.56 Will the medication interfere with my heart tablets/diabetes tablets?

It is important always to check with your doctor or a pharmacist when adding new medication to the ones that you are already taking. This applies to ones bought over the counter or from a health food shop as well as ones that have been prescribed. The motto is 'if in doubt, ask'.

STEROIDS AND LIDOCAINE (LIGNOCAINE)

9.1   Do steroid injections work in OA joints?

Yes. Steroid injections do relieve pain and increase flexibility of joints. These injections may be particularly effective in relieving pain arising from the carpometacarpal joint of the thumb. Some patients obtain months of pain relief when steroids are injected into knee joints. Only a few patients experience transient relief (i.e. less than 3 weeks). Importantly, even this may be significant if the injection can be combined with an exercise programme so that the muscles protecting the joint are built up and these in turn will allow more pain-free flexibility/mobility.

9.2   Which joints respond well to steroid injections in OA?

The classical joints to inject with steroids are the knee joint and the thumb carpometacarpal (CMC) joint. Sometimes the CMC joint will require a course of three injections spaced about 6 weeks apart. Steroid injections are worthwhile trying on any joint affected by OA. A good response is pain relief for greater than 6 weeks, hopefully for more than 3 months; some patients experience pain relief and decreased swelling for much longer, even for years. The principle is to give pain relief so as to allow self-physiotherapy, or a prescribed course of physiotherapy, to build up the muscles, which will protect the injected joint and so allow more pain-free activities.

9.3   Some patients with OA hands have large thick fingers and poor grip. Do they respond to steroid injections?

Yes. Very often injections into the flexor tendon sheaths of the affected fingers return some, if not all, of the patient's finger flexibility. If an injection is given before the fingers have become too immobile, the patient will regain the ability to oppose the finger tips into the palm of the hand. The best example is golf players who are finding gripping the golf club difficult but have not yet given up golf; injections into the flexor sheaths will restore the grip. If the loss of grip has become too disabling, as in the case of the golfer who has given up playing, then it is usually too late for an injection to be effective.

9.4   Do steroid injections have to be given into the knee joint?

Best practice suggests that a better result is obtained if the injection is placed correctly—in this case in the joint. Interestingly, work in Dublin and Nottingham (Jones et al 1993) indicates that we do not enter the knee joint as often as we would expect. The average is around 50%; naturally, some people have a better average than others.

Interestingly, some doctors give repeat injections of a small amount of steroid and larger amounts of lidocaine (lignocaine) into the area of the anserine bursa. This appears to give just as good results as injecting into the joint itself and is useful in patients with extremely large knees, especially those who, for a variety of reasons, are not suitable for total knee replacement. There is no published evidence to support this, only case studies and clinical use.

9.5   Does lidocaine (lignocaine) work when used alone or does it have to be combined with a steroid?

There is little published evidence on the answer to this question (Adebajo et al 1990, Berry et al 1980, Petri et al 1987, Rizk et al 1991, Vecchio et al 1993). It is quite possible that lidocaine will work well on its own; it certainly does when injected into tender/trigger points of fibromyalgia. There is an MRC study underway looking at just this question, but it will be some time before the results are published. In the meantime, it seems expedient to combine steroid and lidocaine in the majority of procedures (*see Q. 9.27*).

9.6   What is the maximum amount of lidocaine (lignocaine) that may be used?

The amount of lidocaine used should not exceed 200 mg (20 mL of 1% or 10 mL of 2% for the average adult). This amount may need to be reduced for smaller patients. The most likely scenarios where doses are excessive are in performing shoulder or trochanteric bursa injections, as well as a few injections into smaller joints. For this reason, when adding lidocaine to steroid, it is advisable to use 1% lidocaine rather than 2% as it gives a wider safety margin (*see Q. 9.7*).

These days it is probably the central nervous side-effects that are the problem rather than the cardiovascular side-effects (*see Qs 9.13 and 9.14*).

9.7   Should 1% or 2% lidocaine (lignocaine) be used?

This is probably personal preference but it should also encompass safety. The maximum dose for the average adult is 200 mg. This is more easily exceeded if 2% lidocaine rather than 1% is used when larger volumes are being injected. It is therefore sensible to use 1% lidocaine when using large volumes for some shoulder injections and trochanteric bursa injections, for example (*see Q. 9.6*). 2% lidocaine may be used for adding to steroid when injecting small joints (*see Q. 9.14*).

9.8   How long do steroid injections take to work?

It all depends on what the injection was given for. Injections into a thumb carpometacarpal joint will usually cause discomfort for 3–4 days then give very good pain relief. Injections into knees give similar results. Some patients get instant relief, but they are often the ones who have had synovial fluid removed from the knee as well as a steroid injection. Other patients will have discomfort for at least a week, followed by a good response. Injections for soft tissue problems may not give as much discomfort as injections into joints, but the response may take up to 3 weeks to occur.

9.9 Are there any differences in potency between hydrocortisone, triamcinolone and methylprednisolone?

Hydrocortisone has always been considered the weakest of the three commonly available injectable steroids. Some therapists use hydrocortisone when they consider that there are greater risks of causing side-effect; for example, when injecting into tendon sheaths, especially in the case of an Achilles or a De Quervain tenosynovitis. Sometimes, hydrocortisone is used if there is a greater than usual risk of fat atrophy in thin skin at the injection site.

There is evidence in the case of children with arthritis that the use of triamcinolone hexacetonide leads to an increased and more prolonged response compared to methylprednisolone. Unfortunately, this formulation (proprietary name Lederspan) is no longer available, although it is possible that this is only a prolonged temporary phenomenon. Triamcinolone acetonide is available; its proprietary name is Adcortyl.

Methylprednisolone has the advantage that it can be combined with lidocaine (lignocaine). This is useful when wishing to reduce the volume of injection fluid.

In essence, the choice comes down to personal preference or even the logistics of supply and storage (*see Q. 9.10*).

9.10 When should hydrocortisone be used?

There are no absolute rules for when any steroid must be used. Use of a particular steroid, with or without lidocaine (lignocaine), is a personal preference. Some therapists prefer hydrocortisone in situations where they consider there are particular risks (e.g. risk of tendon rupture or skin depigmentation). In certain situations, it may be worthwhile assessing the use of lidocaine alone before considering the use of a steroid (*see Q. 9.9*).

9.11 Lidocaine (lignocaine) added to methylprednisolone causes flocculation. Does this matter?

Some purists consider that, when the preparations flocculate, the methylprednisolone loses its full potency. This was one of the reasons why a combined preparation of methylprednisolone and lidocaine was produced (Depo-Medrone with Lidocaine).

In clinical practice, there does not appear to be any problems with potency and efficacy when using methylprednisolone with added lidocaine that has flocculated. Similarly, when further lidocaine is added to Depo-

Medrone with Lidocaine and flocculation occurs, this does not cause problems clinically or decrease efficacy.

9.12 Can lidocaine (lignocaine) be added to Depo-Medrone with Lidocaine?

Yes, although it may cause flocculation. Clinically, this does not seem to be important (*see Q. 9.11*).

9.13 What are the important cardiovascular side-effects of using lidocaine (lignocaine) for joint and soft tissue injections?

Lidocaine is unlikely to give cardiovascular side-effects as it is usually used in relatively small quantities and is not being given as a bolus intravenously. The likely side-effects are bradycardia and hypotension. Importantly, because of the rapid metabolism and elimination of lidocaine, any cardiovascular side-effects are likely to be very transient.

9.14 What are the central nervous side-effects of using lidocaine (lignocaine) for joint and soft tissue injections?

These days, patients travel to see their therapists using all forms of transport and the central nervous side-effects of injections are most important. Lidocaine may cause dizziness, confusion, drowsiness and even paraesthesia. When used for injections and not given as a bolus intravenously, it is unlikely to cause respiratory depression or convulsions.

Prevention of side-effects is obviously most important. Their incidence and severity may be reduced by limiting the amount of lidocaine used at any given session. The total dose of lidocaine should not exceed 200 mg by weight in the average person. This amount should be reduced for frail and more elderly patients.

The practical way of reducing the average dosage is to use 1% lidocaine for injections. This gives 20 mL (200 mg) of 1% lidocaine available for use. The use of 2% lidocaine should be discouraged because, if several sites are to be injected, 10 mL (200 mg) can easily be exceeded. The risks are greatest for the elderly, especially the small and frail.

9.15 What information should be given to a patient after an injection?

Following an injection the patient should be given written information to take away (*see Fig. 9.1*). This information should complement what has already been discussed during the consultation.

9.16 How common is infection after injection of a joint?

The chance of a joint injection causing a joint infection is in the order of 1:77 300 (Seror et al 1999), which indicates that the chance of seeing or

STEROID INJECTIONS

- You have been given a steroid injection today. This has a powerful anti-inflammatory effect on painful tendons, muscles and joints. This effect builds up over three to four days.

- The area may be more painful for a few days. You may need to take one or two tablets of paracetamol, or your usual painkiller, to help the pain. N.B. Follow the instructions on the container or on the leaflet in the box.

- It is important that you follow the instructions that you have been given about exercising the joint.

Are there any complications of having this injection?

There may be a small amount of discomfort. Side-effects are rare but may occur. These include:

- If you experience any pain or discomfort it usually subsides within a few days (see above).
- Some patients experience facial flushing. Do not worry as this usually subsides within a day or two.
- Diabetic patients need to monitor their blood/urine sugars as these may rise. Diet and medication may have to be adjusted for a few days following the injection.
- Some women find that there is some irregularity of the menstrual cycle following the injection. This may be in the form of break-through bleeding or a missed period. If you are concerned, please contact your GP.
- Sometimes the injection fluid can leak back and cause some skin irritation and, on rare occasions, skin thinning.
- Occasionally, the site of the injection can become **infected:** this is extremely **rare**. Signs of developing infection include the area becoming sore and starting to throb after the first 24 hours. Sometimes it will look red and angry. If either of these problems occur, or you are concerned for any reason, then contact a doctor on the same day to check whether treatment is needed.

▲

Fig. 9.1 Example of 'steroid injection notes' for patients.

causing a joint infection is not very high. BUT, with the increasing use of hyaluronan injections, it is possible that swollen, hot joints may be encountered. This is invariably a pseudo-infection, but a full-blown bacterial infection will need to be excluded (*see Q. 9.36*).

9.17 How many injections may be given at one session?

There are no rules. All injections cause some discomfort, with injections into small joints, especially of the feet, producing the most discomfort. The majority of patients will tolerate about seven injections before feeling too much discomfort.

Some knee injections may be extremely painful and it is often worthwhile, in apprehensive patients, using a local anaesthetic first. This approach is recommended for repeat knee injections (e.g. when administering a course of hyaluronans).

9.18 How soon can an injection be repeated?

There are two clinical pictures that this question relates to:

- The patient who has had a poor response and is requesting another injection: is it appropriate?
- The patient who has had a good or adequate response to the injection: when is it sensible to give another?

The practical answer to the first scenario is that a wait of 3–4 weeks seems sensible and then the patient may be reviewed. All patients vary and a further injection may be appropriate for one patient but not for another. For example, OA of the carpometacarpal joint of the thumb responds very well to steroid injections, but some patients will require a course of three injections before obtaining an acceptable response.

The best example of the second scenario is patients with knee OA who had a good response to the steroid injection. The first injection usually gives increased mobility and 6–8 weeks of pain relief. Hopefully, a second injection will be effective for 3–4 months. Subsequent injections, given every 4 months, will usually give an excellent clinical response. Some patients will mobilize so well that their quadriceps improve to allow less frequent injections.

9.19 Is it true that injections should not be given into a specific joint more than three or four times a year?

 This is a practical rule, based upon good clinical practice. It is unlikely that three or four steroid injections into the same joint over 1 year will do any permanent damage, but every time an injection is given the therapist should always be thinking if this is an appropriate way to manage the condition and asking if the diagnosis is still the same. Remember, that this 'rule' applies to a particular joint, so that other joints may still be injected, but, again, apply the same principles.

9.20 Is there evidence to show that steroid injections may cause a Charcot joint?

 One of the folk myths says that too many steroid injections into a joint can cause a Charcot joint picture, but, from reviewing the early reports, there is no conclusive evidence to support this.

9.21 What type of technique should be used when performing joint injections?

 A no-touch technique is the best. The important principles are to decrease the bacterial risks/load. Use one needle to draw up the injection and another to inject the patient. Do not use a finger to guide the needle. Remember that the skin and joint capsule are the tissues that have pain fibres.

Synovial fluid can transmit the human immunodeficiency virus (HIV), so the advice is to wear gloves.

9.22 Some doctors insist on the patient resting a joint for 24 h after injection. Is this important?

There is some evidence from patients with RA (rheumatoid arthritis) that resting for 24 h in bed retains the injected steroid in the joint for longer. Unfortunately, in today's hectic world this is not really practical. Nowadays, the advice is simply to be sensible and not to overuse the injected joint for the next few days.

9.23 Following an injection the joint may be painful. How long does this usually last?

This discomfort, even pain, may last 3 or 4 days and generally clears totally after about 5 days. It is important to discuss this with patients and mention it in the steroid injection leaflet that is given to patients.

9.24 How important is it to make sure that the injection goes into the joint?

For the best results an injection should be given into the correct place. There is some evidence to support this but it is not overwhelming.

Exact placing of hyaluronan injections is more important than exact placing of steroid injections. Hyaluronans are only likely to work if placed in the joint, steroid injections are assumed to diffuse into the joint if placed outside it.

9.25   **What is the best placement of tennis and golfer's elbow injections?**

The best results are obtained by directing the needle down onto and into the periosteum. The injection should raise the periosteum; i.e. the injection is in essence producing a 'medical tendon slide', similar to the surgical operation. In some patients the pain of the epicondylitis is so severe that it is difficult to 'reach' the periosteum. Leaving the steroid at the periosteum will give moderate pain relief, usually allowing an accurate injection, if required, 3–6 weeks later.

9.26   **To relieve knee pain caused by OA, do injections have to be given into the joint or are there other places to inject?**

The teaching is to inject the knee joint with steroid and lidocaine (lignocaine). Some knees are so large that entering the joint cannot be done with absolute certainty. Even so, these patients often obtain great relief. This has led some therapists to inject outside the joint, usually on the medial aspect in the region of the anserine bursa. This is at the point of maximum tenderness on the medial aspect (probably on the acupuncture spleen 9 line) and is usually found by the patient placing the hand on the knee at the maximum point of tenderness, which will be found just below the patient's thumb.

An injection of steroid plus lidocaine, or lidocaine alone, into this area will often give excellent results. This procedure may be used to great effect for patients who are on warfarin, are obese or too great a cardiac or anaesthetic risk for total knee replacement.

9.27   **How important is the steroid in the injected fluid?**

It is assumed that the steroid is the important ingredient in the injection, but there is an on-going debate as to whether or not this is true. For instance, some patients with OA knees respond well to lidocaine (lignocaine) alone when injected into the medial aspect of the knee. Patients with tender points (sometimes called trigger points) over their shoulders and neck respond for weeks, even months, to lidocaine alone.

Whether inflamed joints would respond as well to lidocaine alone compared to steroid alone has not been investigated. The MRC has recently given a grant for a clinical trial of lidocaine alone against steroid alone in subacromial bursitis: the results will be of great interest (*see Q. 9.5*).

9.28   **How important is the lidocaine (lignocaine) in the injected fluid?**

This is not as simple a question as it first appears; nor is the answer (*see Box 9.1*).

BOX 9.1 How important is lidocaine (lignocaine) in the injected fluid?

- The lidocaine is not there to make the injection less painful.
- The lidocaine will help the therapist decide if the injection has been placed accurately. For instance, 5 min after an injection into the subacromial bursa for a painful arc of abduction, the patient should be able to perform the arc without much discomfort.
- The lidocaine acts as a diluent and may decrease the risk of superficial skin atrophy if there is leakage of the injection fluid back along the needle track.
- Using a larger volume may allow less pinpoint accuracy but give the same results as a smaller volume accurately placed.
- Lidocaine is a local anaesthetic, but it also has a central effect on pain which lasts much longer, possibly weeks. This may explain its beneficial effects when used alone (e.g. for tender point injections) (*see Q. 9.5*).

9.29 Patients with OA hips may have additional pain from a trochanteric bursitis. Is this worth an injection?

Yes. Pain from a superficial or deep trochanteric bursitis is always worth treating with a steroid injection. Usually, there is a remarkable reduction in pain and a corresponding improvement in mobility. The injection may need to be repeated as the underlying problem remains—i.e. the OA hip joint causing a change in gait. Trochanteric bursitis may occur after hip replacement; this will respond to injections, but it would be sensible to refer the patient for further physiotherapy to check that the gait has returned to normal.

9.30 How long does the beneficial effect of steroid/lidocaine (lignocaine) injections last?

Most patient responses fall into three broad bands:

- Patients who only benefit for between a few days and 3 weeks.
- Patients who benefit for 3–4 months.
- Patients who benefit for a remarkably long period (years; a response of 3–5 years is not uncommon).

HYALURONANS

9.31 What are hyaluronan injections?

Hyaluronan is found in synovial fluid and is secreted by the synovial lining. It normally has a high molecular weight, giving it a high viscosity.

Hyaluronan acts as a lubricant and a shock-absorber and is said to help in joint repair as well as joint protection. In OA, the viscosity falls; injecting hyaluronan increases this viscosity back towards normal levels. This seems good in theory but hyaluronan is cleared rapidly from the synovial fluid into the general circulation; this is the manufacturer's explanation as to why a course of 3–5 injections should to be given at weekly intervals. There could be other explanations (*see Q. 9.32*) and there are other theories as to why hyaluronan works in OA joints.

9.32   There are many preparations of hyaluronans. What is the rationale in choosing the one to use?

Most preparations are delivered as a course of 2-mL injections. Between three and five injections are given at either a week or 2 weeks apart. There is one preparation for which only one injection of 6 mL is needed, but the evidence of its efficacy over saline is not very strong. It may be necessary to enter the joint when injecting hyaluronan for it to be effective. This may explain why there is a greater efficacy in the trials using a course of injections. This is backed up by evidence of hyaluronans being injected into hips under ultrasound guidance; the preliminary results look very promising.

The problem with courses of injections is that patients require to be seen more often, which is time-consuming and expensive. For this reason alone, it could be said that the shorter the course the better as long as there are at least three injections, as the evidence suggests that only 50% of injections enter the joint. The alternative answer is to inject under ultrasound control if this is feasible.

9.33   When injecting knees, how often does the needle enter the joint space?

The evidence from the two studies that have looked at the accuracy of injections concluded that the answer is that 50% of injections enter the knee joint. There are no available studies on smaller joints. If ultrasound is used to help guide the injection, then the success rate should be 100% but it is probably in the region of 75%. This is because there are two ways of using ultrasound: one using the transducer in real time and one that uses the ultrasound to measure the distance/depth and position that the needle needs to be placed in order to obtain joint entry. The latter is the common way, as the former requires sterile procedures and an assistant; otherwise, the therapist has only one hand for the transducer and one for the needle and syringe.

9.34 How important is it to deliver the hyaluronan into the joint space?

It is very important in order to obtain an excellent or good result. Because hyaluronans have a very high molecular weight, they are unlikely to diffuse into the joint if placed outside the joint capsule. Retrospective analysis of case studies of hyaluronan injections gives a success rate of about 50%; this increases to over 70% if the injections are ultrasound-'enhanced'.

9.35 Are there problems if hyaluronan is delivered outside the joint capsule?

This question has not been fully evaluated. Some manufacturers consider that there is a higher incidence of side-effects if the hyaluronan is delivered outside the joint capsule. These side-effects range from mild injection-site reactions, through joint effusion to pseudo-infection. The joint effusion in the pseudo-infections looks like pus and does have large numbers of macrophages on microscopy. The essential point is that these effusions do not grow organisms, but infection MUST be excluded. The problem for people managing these patients is NOT to treat as a joint infection until proved, as some drug regimens also have severe side-effects (*see* Q. *9.36*).

The majority of side-effects caused by hyaluronans occur within the first 48 h.

9.36 A very small number of patients develop a severe, painful effusion after a hyaluronan injection. How should this be managed?

These problems usually occur within the first few days following an injection of hyaluronan.

SMALL EFFUSION PLUS SOME DISCOMFORT

Patients should be advised to take their pain medication for the discomfort. The effusion rarely needs drainage unless the discomfort is severe.

SEVERE DISCOMFORT PLUS EFFUSION

These patients have a tense knee and it appears that the effusion plays a large part in the pain. Importantly, the effusion may only be around 20 mL in volume but the pain relief produced by removing it is excellent. The effusion is invariably straw-coloured. If it is not, then samples of aspirate should be sent off for culture to exclude infection.

LARGE EFFUSION WITH KNEE PAIN

Most large effusions should be drained. This gives good pain relief and allows fluid to be sent for culture to exclude infection. The result is rarely positive. The fluid is usually straw-coloured and sterile.

Sometimes there is a recurrence of the effusion and aspiration needs to be repeated. The discomfort from this rapid accumulation of fluid may be severe and it is this factor that should dictate whether or not to aspirate.

NSAIDs/COX-2 inhibitors do not appear to stop accumulation of the fluid, but of course they should give good pain relief.

Removing fluid and injecting a steroid does not appear to stop the re-accumulation of fluid. Some therapists do suggest this course of action, but simple aspiration alone certainly gives good pain relief.

PSEUDO-INFECTION EFFUSIONS WITH KNEE PAIN

This type of effusion is rarely seen, but it is a great worry when it is. The pain and discomfort are no different from the large straw-coloured effusion, but in this case the fluid looks just like frank pus (yellow/grey/green). The knee joint is warm but not as hot as one would expect if this was a true infection; nor is the patient ill, although they do have severe pain.

It is essential to send the fluid for culture and microscopy. Importantly, do not treat for infection solely on a laboratory report of macrophages. Treating inappropriately with gentamicin, for example, may lead to worse side-effects than those caused by the hyaluronan.

Removing the fluid alone gives adequate pain relief. Some patients will require analgesia as well. The joint does not require wash-out or surgical debridement. If medical staff are not informed about the possibility that the pseudo-infection effusion has been caused by hyaluronan, there is a risk of inappropriate treatments being carried out. Thankfully, this type of effusion is rare.

9.37   If a patient has a reactive effusion following hyaluronan injection, does this reaction stop the hyaluronan working?

No. Very often patients who have a reaction obtain a long-term good response.

9.38   How soon do hyaluronans start to work?

Steroid injections, or even simple joint aspiration, will give almost instant pain relief. Hyaluronan takes much longer to give pain relief and increased mobility. The time is measured in weeks rather than days. From a practical aspect, if the patient has not had any significant improvement within 3 months, then they have not responded to the course.

9.39   How long does hyaluronan work for?

There is no clear-cut answer to this question, but it is expected that patients will gain improvements of knee function, with less pain, for over 1 year. Studies show that patients obtain relief for at least 6 months. The length of the improvement may depend upon the state of the knee joint and other clinical aspects of the patient (*see Q. 9.40*).

9.40   Which patients with knee OA should be offered hyaluronan?

A straightforward question but not an easy one to answer. Patients with clinically moderate OA appear to respond well to hyaluronan injections. In practice, it is wise to try a steroid injection first as some patients respond favourably. The accuracy of the sighting of the steroid injection is not as critical as for hyaluronans and only one injection is required.

Patients with an effusion or severe knee OA tend not to respond as well to hyaluronan, but it may need to be tried if other forms of therapy have not helped or the patient has other medical problems which rule out a total knee replacement. In this group of patients, the response is 30–40%. There is the possibility that side-effects to hyaluronan injections are more common in these patients.

9.41   When, in OA, should hyaluronan injections be performed to obtain the best results?

Both clinical studies and clinical use suggest that hyaluronans should be used when patients have moderate OA of the knee. This can be assessed clinically. Patients with moderate OA have knee pain that is intrusive/disruptive in a significant proportion of daily activities. The level of function impairment is that some recreational, leisure or work activities are significantly disrupted and some help or aid (e.g. sorbothane insoles) is required, without which these activities are impossible.

These patients will have both active and passive joint movements that are slow, restricted and painful; there may be a small effusion. X-rays of weight-bearing knees will show definite joint space narrowing, as well as osteophytes, and there may well be sclerosis and changes in subchondral bone.

9.42   Is it worthwhile using hyaluronan for patients who require total knee replacement but are medically unfit for the operation?

Yes (*see Q. 9.40*). The main problem is that only 30–40% of patients respond, but this may well be acceptable in this group of patients. In these cases, it would be worthwhile injecting under ultrasound to increase the chances of the injection being sited within the knee joint.

9.43 Is hyaluronan used only on knee joints?

There are on-going studies looking at the use of hyaluronans in small joints such as the thumb carpometacarpal joint. It is likely that only one injection will be used. For hip joints it may be necessary to inject under ultrasound control.

9.44 Can steroids be injected into joints that have had hyaluronan injected?

Yes, there is no known contraindication to injecting steroids after hyaluronan injections have been given.

9.45 How many injections of hyaluronan need to be given?

The licence for the majority of the hyaluronan products is for a course of 3–5 injections at weekly intervals. These products have been on the market for some time so that clinical usage has produced variations from the licence. The manufacturers have clinical studies looking at many variations:

■ Injection under ultrasound control
■ Single injections of different volumes
■ Repeat injections for 'need' rather than at a fixed-time interval.

Until these studies are completed the best advice is to use hyaluronan according to the licence indications.

9.46 When can a further course of hyaluronan be given?

If the patient has had a good response to the hyaluronan injection, then this can be repeated as necessary. There is no formula for predicting when the patient will relapse; studies suggest that the average time is 6 months, but this can vary from 4 to 18 months.

9.47 What are the contraindications for hyaluronan?

There are a few contraindications:
■ Severely inflamed joints
■ Infected joints
■ Venous stasis
■ Lymphatic stasis
■ Sensitivity to product derivatives.

PQ PATIENT QUESTIONS

9.48 I am told that my injected joint may be painful and sore following the injection. How long will the pain and soreness last?

Some patients have no pain and soreness. Others will have some pain and soreness which will usually last for a few days, typically 3 or 4, but it may last up to a week.

9.49 If my injected joint is painful, what can I take for the pain?

If you need to take something for the pain, usually a couple of paracetamol or co-codamol will give relief. You may take similar medication that you have been prescribed for pain relief.

9.50 If my injected joint is painful and sore, at what stage should I phone for advice?

You should seek advice when you are concerned about the situation. This would usually be if the joint became hot or very warm and if the pain was increasing rather than decreasing. Certainly, if you felt ill or unwell it would be sensible to ask for advice.

9.51 How can I tell if my joint is infected?

The classical symptoms are:

■ A very hot or warm area around the joint
■ This area may be red
■ The joint will be painful and becoming more painful
■ You may feel ill or unwell.

If these symptoms do occur you should certainly seek advice. This picture is extremely rare but do not let that put you off phoning if you are concerned.

9.52 What can I do to make the injection (effects) last longer?

Initially, that is in the first 24–48 h, do not overuse the joint; this allows the injection to stay in the joint itself. After 48 h you should gradually increase the use of the injected joint(s). This will improve the range of movement and, most importantly, strengthen the muscles that move the joint. The principle is that the larger and stronger the muscles, the more they will protect the joint and so lessen the pain. This applies to all joints, but in particular to the knee joint. Do your own physiotherapy exercises and build up the quadriceps muscles around the knee.

Pharmacological management 5: Glucosamine, other drug therapies and the future

10

PQ PATIENT QUESTIONS

GLUCOSAMINE

10.1 What is glucosamine and how does it work?

Glucosamine is a complex aminosugar. It is a normal constituent of the glycosaminoglycans that occur naturally in cartilage matrix and synovial fluid. When taken orally, it is absorbed and distributed to the tissues of joints.

10.2 What is the current evidence for the effectiveness of glucosamine?

Reginster et al (2001) reported a double-blind randomized placebo-controlled trial with 3-year follow-up in patients with mild to moderate OA of the knee; 212 patients were enrolled and randomly assigned to glucosamine sulphate at a dose of 1500 mg or matching placebo. This study looked at two separate aspects: structural changes within the joint and symptoms of osteoarthritis.

The primary outcome measure for structural change was the mean joint space width of the medial compartment of the tibiofemoral joint measured radiologically using a standardized technique. The primary outcome measure for symptoms of OA was the WOMAC scale (*see Appendix 1*) using the visual analogue version.

Results showed a progressive and significant narrowing of joint space in 106 patients on placebo, but there was no significant joint space loss in the 106 patients on glucosamine. Symptoms as assessed by the WOMAC score showed improvement in patients on glucosamine, with slight worsening in patients on placebo. There were no differences in safety or early withdrawal between the groups.

Although the results of this study look promising, the authors state that it is not yet possible to tell whether the joint space narrowing detected will be of clinical importance in the longer term and that further long-term studies are required.

Hughes & Carr (2002) reported a randomized placebo-controlled trial with 80 patients with OA of knee over 6 months. This was a pragmatic trial including the sort of patients presenting routinely to their GP with pain from OA knee. Patients were allowed to continue NSAIDs (non-steroidal anti-inflammatory drugs) and or analgesics already prescribed and encouraged to avoid changing dose or preparation during the study. The primary outcome measure was the patient's assessment of pain in the affected knee. In this study, analysis showed no difference between glucosamine and placebo in the primary outcome measure—namely, patients' global pain assessment—although there was a small but statistically significant improvement in knee flexion. It was therefore concluded that glucosamine was no more effective than placebo in modifying pain in patients with a wide range of pain severity.

10.3 What might account for the difference between the two studies, each of which used the same dose of glucosamine of 1500 mg per day?

Patients in the smaller study (Hughes & Carr 2002) had radiologically and symptomatically more severe OA than in Reginster's trial (2001), and it may be that glucosamine is more effective in milder OA.

10.4 Are there any other studies looking at the effectiveness of glucosamine?

A meta-analysis of double-blind randomized controlled trials lasting 4 weeks or more looking at glucosamine and chondroitin in OA was published in 2000 (McAlindon et al 2000). This analysis suggested that, although moderate to large effects were noted for symptoms of OA, issues involving quality and publication bias probably exaggerated the results.

10.5 What is chondroitin and how does it work?

Chondroitin sulphate is a proteoglycan that occurs naturally within the cartilage matrix. The chondroitin sold as a supplement has a bovine origin. There is less evidence for the effectiveness of chondroitin sulphate than there is for glucosamine in the treatment of OA. Chondroitin is sometimes sold as an individual product although it is often sold combined with glucosamine.

10.6 Is the effect of glucosamine dose-dependent?

Both of the above studies were undertaken with a dose of 1500 mg glucosamine per day, and there is as yet no real evidence that lower doses are effective. It is important to tell patients that the results discussed above apply only to this dose as glucosamine is sold in many different doses and formulations.

10.7 Does glucosamine have any side-effects?

Neither the Reginster et al (2001) study nor the Hughes & Carr (2002) study found any difference in side-effects between glucosamine and placebo. There is a theoretical risk of increased blood sugar in diabetic patients but this has not proved to be a problem.

10.8 What is the evidence for disease-modifying properties of glucosamine?

In the trial reported by Reginster et al (2001) there was no significant joint space loss in patients on glucosamine over 3 years, whereas patients on placebo showed progressive joint space narrowing.

10.9 Is glucosamine cost-effective?

Glucosamine can be bought in bulk over the Internet and in high street pharmacies and health food shops. It is relatively inexpensive compared with the costs of analgesics, NSAIDs and other non-pharmacological interventions for OA knee.

10.10 Can glucosamine be prescribed on FP10?

Glucosamine is an unlicensed medicine and, although some doctors do prescribe it on FP10, most prescribing advisors would suggest that it should not be given in this way. Glucosamine comes under the category of 'pay and report', thus practitioners prescribing glucosamine on FP10 may be required to justify their actions. As there is evidence from randomized controlled trials for the effectiveness of glucosamine this should not present a problem, but in most areas it may be prudent to check with the local Trust before prescribing.

10.11 Should glucosamine be given alone or can it be taken together with analgesics and NSAIDs?

There are no known interactions for glucosamine and therefore no reason why it should not be co-prescribed with NSAIDs and analgesics.

OTHER DRUG THERAPIES

10.12 Apart from NSAIDs/COX-2 inhibitors, analgesics, injections and topical preparations are there any other drug strategies that can be employed to treat OA?

Low-dose amitriptyline taken in the evening may be a useful adjunct to analgesic and anti-inflammatory therapy. At a dose of 10–25 mg it has really no action as an antidepressant but seems to enhance the analgesic action of other drugs. To avoid a hangover effect in the morning it is often best taken around 7–8 p.m. rather than at bedtime. If a tricyclic antidepressant is contraindicated, then a selective serotonin re-uptake inhibitor at low dose may be preferable. Remember that patients who are severely disabled by OA may become clinically depressed and may require full-dose antidepressant therapy.

10.13 Is there any place for the use of opiate controlled drugs in the management of OA?

Patients with severe OA may suffer very considerable pain when the joint deteriorates with almost total loss of cartilage. In these patients, joint replacement surgery can remove this severe pain, but the period of time prior to the operation can be very distressing. Strong opiate drugs (controlled drugs) are sometimes used at this time, with the usual caveats of contraindications, interactions and, of course, dependency. Postoperatively following the joint replacement, the pain relief experienced by these patients is usually very considerable and there is then no need for further prescriptions of these strong analgesics. These strong drugs may also have a place in patients with severely destroyed joints and for whom surgery is contraindicated or refused by the patient. Drugs such as pentazocine, fentanyl, oxycodone, buprenorphine and some morphine-based compounds are occasionally used in this way. Some of these drugs are licensed for severe chronic pain; others are only licensed for cancer and postoperative pain. Buprenorphine was recently launched as a matrix patch which offers pain relief for up to 72 h and is licensed both for cancer pain and for chronic severe non-malignant pain. Although these drugs should certainly not be used routinely in the management of OA, there may be a place for their occasional use in patients such as those indicated above for whom all other forms of pain relief have failed.

10.14 What drugs are recommended as gastric protection when required with NSAID therapy?

Proton pump inhibitors (PPI) and misoprostol are both licensed for the healing of NSAID-associated gastric and duodenal ulceration. H_2-receptor antagonists may be effective for NSAID-associated duodenal ulcers only. Treatment with misoprostol may be limited by diarrhoea and colic, is contraindicated in pregnancy and best avoided in women of childbearing age. PPIs are also best avoided during pregnancy and lactation. NICE guidance suggests that in high-risk patients for whom an anti-inflammatory drug is essential and a COX-2 inhibitor is contraindicated, a standard NSAID should be used together with a PPI.

THE FUTURE: POTENTIAL NEW DRUGS FOR OA

10.15 Are there any potential new pharmacological therapies to treat the symptoms of OA?

There appear to be two separate pathways from arachidonic acid to the production of inflammatory mediators. One pathway is mediated by cyclo-oxygenase (COX), to produce prostaglandins. COX-1 mediates the production of the prostaglandins that protect gastric mucosa and kidney function; COX-2 facilitates the production of inflammatory mediators. In a second pathway, arachidonic acid is metabolized by the enzyme 5-lipoxygenase, resulting in the production of the leukotriene LTB_4, among others, which also contributes to the production of inflammation. Thus a drug which inhibits both COX and 5-lipoxygenase may reduce gastric toxicity while at the same time producing increased anti-inflammatory activity and therefore greater efficacy. Looking at the situation from another direction, molecules that can replace inflammatory mediators as opposed to blocking their production could also have a place in modulating inflammation. Nitric oxide appears to have this ability and has been shown to produce gastroduodenal protection in a similar way to prostaglandins. Drugs are being developed to donate nitric oxide and are called cyclo-oxygenase-inhibiting nitric oxide donors. Other drugs (e.g. licofelone) are being developed to inhibit 5-lipoxygenase. Both of these new classes of drugs show a promising reduction in gastrointestinal toxicity and studies are awaited looking at efficacy.

Bisphosphonates, which are currently used in the management of osteoporosis, may have a place as disease-modifying drugs in OA. Research to investigate this possibility is on-going. If the results are positive, the exciting possibility arises of having one drug to treat two common degenerative conditions.

10.16 What is the future in terms of prevention of OA?

It is thought that the pathological changes seen in OA result from an imbalance between catabolic and anabolic processes. The catabolic processes are induced by the cytokines, interleukin 1 (IL-1) and tumour necrosis factor (TNF), which are involved much earlier in the inflammatory cascade than cyclo-oxygenase (*see Fig. 10.1*). If the actions of these cytokines are blocked, this may prevent cartilage breakdown. Diacerein is a new compound which antagonizes the synthesis and activity of IL-1 and may act as a disease-modifying drug in OA. As well as inhibiting IL-1, diacerein seems to inhibit other pro-inflammatory cytokines. As well as an inhibitory role, diacerein also seems to have a role in the synthesis of some of the constituents of cartilage, such as collagen and proteoglycans. Diacerein has no inhibitory effect on the synthesis of prostaglandins and therefore, unlike NSAIDs, shows no gastroduodenal toxicity. Clinical trials of diacerein are on-going and early results suggest that this oral drug may be effective in relieving the symptoms of OA as well as showing good tolerability and virtually no gastroduodenal problems. If diacerein is also shown to have a disease-modifying effect, as animal studies suggest, then this drug promises to be very useful in the management of OA.

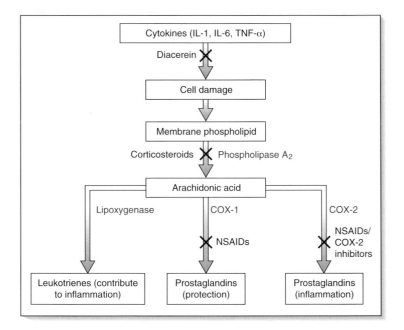

Fig. 10.1 Simplified version of part of the inflammatory cascade showing sites of action of diacerein and corticosteroids. IL-1, interleukin 1; IL-6, interleukin 6; TNF-α, tumour necrosis factor-α.

Other potential disease-modifying agents include those that inhibit matrix metalloprotease (MMP). Tetracycline and the semi-synthetic forms doxycycline and minocycline show considerable activity against MMP and research is on-going. So, although, apart from glucosamine there is as yet no specific disease-modifying drug for OA, there are certainly several promising drugs in the development stages.

PQ PATIENT QUESTIONS

10.17 My friend takes glucosamine tablets from the health food shop for her arthritis. I asked my doctor if I could get them on prescription but he said that I had to buy them. Is it worth my while buying them?

Evidence is accumulating that glucosamine may have a place in slowing progression in knee osteoarthritis. As yet, studies have not been published for the effect of glucosamine on other joints. If you have OA of your knees you certainly should consider buying glucosamine. If you have arthritis in other joints it might be worth trying it to see if it helps. The amount used in the studies was one 500-mg tablet taken three times daily.

10.18 Should I try the new 'drugs' that my doctor is suggesting?

You certainly should discuss your worries and concerns about this issue with your doctor. He/she should know more about the drugs and the likely benefits than your friends.

10.19 Will taking tablets make my joints better?

If your pain is relieved and you become more mobile, then you should build up the muscles around the affected joints. These muscles will protect your joints so it is worthwhile undertaking your own physiotherapy to increase muscle strength. This should help slow down the arthritic process and may well lead to some repair. We must remember that we are not bits of metal that can only wear away and rust; we are living beings and have repair mechanisms and processes going on and we need to encourage them.

At present, we do not have any drugs that arrest arthritis. There are some in development. Glucosamine has been shown to improve knee joints to some extent.

Surgical management: What options are there?

11.1 Does a previous menisectomy always cause OA in later life?

 Not always, but even a partial menisectomy is a risk factor for later development of OA knee; 50% of patients will develop an X-ray diagnosis of OA. The situation is worse for elite athletes, especially football players, as they often have cruciate ligament damage, which gives a greater risk of developing OA (Negret et al 1994, Roos et al 1998).

11.2 Does a menisectomy in one knee increase the risk of OA in both knees in later life?

Yes (*see also Q. 11.1*). Both knees have an increased risk of developing OA following menisectomy. The particular meniscus that is removed or operated upon has an influence on later development of OA. The lateral meniscus is less likely to sustain damage, but if this is removed there is an increased risk of developing OA than if the medial meniscus is removed.

11.3 Can a patient with OA knees develop meniscal problems?

Yes. A sudden deterioration of a patient's OA knee may not be solely due to a flare. The increased pain and effusion can be from a meniscal injury caused by twisting during an activity or hobby. The key to making the diagnosis is the presence of an effusion, and the fact that the pain and effusion do not settle as would be expected if it was an OA flare.

11.4 What knee injuries give an increased risk of OA?

The obvious injuries that are likely to give rise to OA later in life are fractures, especially ones that involve joint surfaces or fractures that are not 'repaired' to give normal alignment so that the joint is stressed. Any joint that is unstable or moves 'too far', as occurs in patients with hypermobility (double-jointedness), is more likely to develop OA. The most common example is loss of anterior cruciate ligament integrity. The knee joint will degenerate even if the cartilage is not involved. Our understanding of these issues has been advanced by quality studies involving elite athletes and professional footballers in particular.

The best protection is to have quality quadriceps giving stability to the knee joint. Unfortunately, as people advance in years, the muscles become weaker and the joints less stable; they are therefore more prone to injuries that may lead to OA or accelerate the process. This process is often called secondary OA, especially when it is seen in people under the age of 45.

The less obvious injuries leading to OA are discussed in *Qs 11.1 and 11.2*.

11.5 Why do patients develop effusions in knee joints?

Usually effusions occur following an injury or because the joint has developed an inflammatory arthritis.

Post-traumatic effusions of knee joints usually require aspiration to see whether there is blood present as this would indicate a more severe form of damage (e.g. to the cruciate ligaments). The joint is usually warm and boggy and, if there is enough fluid to cause tension, this will also cause severe pain.

A synovial effusion is fairly common in OA and signifies that the joint cartilage is damaged. The amount of fluid can vary from minimal to extremely large volumes. Large volumes tend to be seen in severely damaged knees.

NB: In a sports person the presence of an effusion should alert us to suspect a meniscal injury. An effusion will also cause wasting of the quadriceps in a remarkably short space of time.

11.6 When should an effusion be drained?

Drainage of an effusion will give pain relief and often increased mobility. This is true of both large and small effusions. In practice, removal of over 5 mL of synovial fluid from an OA knee will often give immediate pain relief. This will lessen the pain and encourage mobility, so allowing strengthening of the quadriceps.

11.7 What operations can be performed by arthroscopy?

The usual operations performed by arthroscopy are:

■ Debridement
■ Menisectomy
■ Cruciate ligament repair.

Arthroscopy is also used for chondrocyte transplantation and similar research procedures in order to repair isolated chondral defects after traumatic injury.

11.8 Which patients should be referred to orthopaedic surgeons?

Put simply, patients who because of their arthritis:

■ Can't sleep
■ Can't walk
■ Can't work.

The primary care team should be referring patients whom the surgeon would wish to operate upon. These are the patients at the

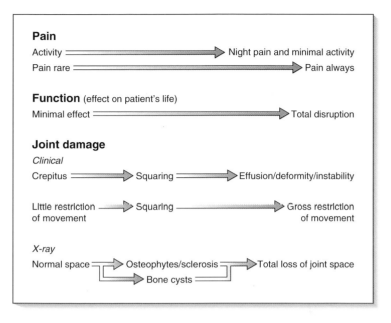

Fig. 11.1 Relationship of pain, function and joint damage with X-ray changes, although a good history and clinical evaluation will determine which patient requires referral rather than relying on an X-ray. From Hosie G, Dickson J 2000 Managing osteoarthritis in primary care (Blackwell Science) with permission.

severe end of the scale for pain, functional disability and structural joint damage (*see Fig. 11.1*).

Pain is the most important parameter, and evidence suggests that if the pain becomes too severe and becomes chronic then the postoperative results are not as good, as some chronic pain persists (Fortin et al 1999, Nilsdotter et al 2002)

11.9 Is joint debridement worthwhile?

Probably not. A recent exemplary trial divided patients into three groups (60 per group):

■ Placebo
■ Lavage
■ Debridement.

Patients were under 75, fulfilled the American College of Rheumatology criteria for osteoarthritis and had a pain score of 40 mm or greater on a 100-mm scale. Patients were followed for 2 years. No outcome showed any difference between placebo and the two active treatments.

Primary care teams should take this evidence on board and be highly selective, as this trial certainly shows that lavage and debridement is not a panacea for all (Moseley et al 2002).

11.10 Which joints respond well to arthroplasty?

In hip and knee joints, arthroplasty has been a resounding success and transformed patients' lives. Shoulder arthroplasty has relieved pain but not improved movement and function. Ankle arthroplasty appears to be good but mostly performed for patients with rheumatoid arthritis (RA). Arthroplasty of smaller joints has not shown the excellent results seen with the large joints. Severe thumb and big toe OA do not respond well to arthroplasty; arthrodesis and osteotomy give better results (*see Q. 11.20*).

11.11 How long should hip and knee arthroplasty last?

At least 10 years and probably 15–20 years. The figures are 90% success rate at 10 years and 75% functioning well at 15 years. These figures definitely apply to hip arthroplasty and probably for knees as well. The 5-year figures for knee are, in fact, better than those for hips. This success rate seems to be slow in influencing the public and the medical profession, as there is still less enthusiasm for this operation compared to hips. The best statistics come from Sweden (*see Fig. 11.2*).

11.12 Which factor, pain or age, should influence the decision whether to refer a patient for arthroplasty?

Pain should be the over-riding factor, not age. If the pain is severe and the patient can't sleep, can't walk, can't work (*see Q. 11.8*), then he or she should be referred and an X-ray taken of the affected joint.

Age should not be a factor. Moreover, there is accumulating evidence suggesting that lengthy waiting times for older patients have a negative effect on the quality of life following an arthroplasty. This is likely to be related to continuing deterioration of the muscles around the affected joint. It is much harder for elderly patients to re-build muscle strength.

11.13 What is the commonest complication of arthroplasty today?

Deep vein thrombosis is the commonest complication, but modern management has greatly reduced this (*see Q. 11.14*). Approximately 10% of patients suffer deep vein thrombosis and 1% suffer pulmonary embolism.

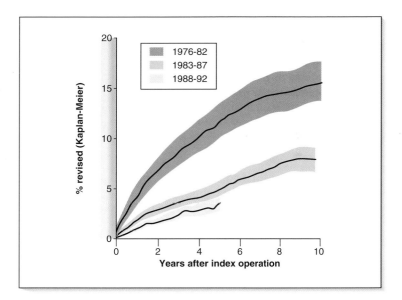

▲

Fig. 11.2 Decreasing revision rates with modern procedures and surgical techniques. From Brandt et al 1998 with permission.

11.14 What factors/prophylaxis have reduced arthroplasty complications?

See Box 11.1.

11.15 What are the revision and complication rates of arthroplasty?

The Swedish National Arthroplasty Register for Hips gives a revision rate for infection of 0.6% at 10 years. About half of this figure is caused by haematogenous spread from other foci (e.g. urinary tract, lungs, gallbladder or dental abscess).

The other half is from 'intra-operative' contamination causing early infection after operation or delayed infection. The patient will not be pain-free, the ESR (erythrocyte sedimentation rate) will be raised and there may be a low-grade fever.

The commonest cause of revision is from loosening; this is around 10% at 10 years.

> **BOX 11.1 Factors that have helped reduce the complications of arthroplasty**
>
> ■ Early mobilization
> ■ Improved surgical techniques
> ■ Prophylactic anticoagulation
> ■ Peri-operative antibiotics
> ■ Critical appraisal of trials for new joint designs
> ■ Hospital and surgeon arthroplasty registers that collate statistics

Often it is the local complications that influence patients and even their medical advisors. Hip operations occasionally damage blood vessels and nerves. The sciatic nerve may be damaged if the operation is combined with hip lengthening. Fractures of the greater trochanter, shaft and acetabulum are more common when uncemented prostheses are used (said to be over 2%). These usually heal well.

Dislocation, especially if recurrent, is distressing for patients and carers. The rate is reported as 0.5–5%. A similar rate is given for trochanteric problems and also for heterotopic bone formation. These groups of problems may seriously reduce mobility.

The knee has often undergone previous operations to the joint before an arthroplasty, so there may be other skin incisions which can affect healing. The joint is nearer the surface and if too large an implant is used there is a greater risk of capsular dehiscence and therefore a risk of deep infection.

Similar problems can affect the patella ligament; incorrect articulation may also be a problem and lead to subluxation and dislocation of the patella. Patients will find the new knee weak and unreliable.

Around 20% of revisions are due to instability and other mechanical factors. Loosening of components, especially the tibial, accounts for 50% of revisions. The revision rate for deep infection is below 1% at 10 years; if it is assumed that at 10 years the revision rate is 10%, then deep infection accounts for less than 10% of this.

11.16 What is an osteotomy?

This is a wedge resection; a piece of bone is removed to change the distribution of the loads on a joint (*see Fig. 11.3*). The aim is to reduce the stresses on the most severely affected areas of the joint and transfer them to areas with more articular cartilage.

11.17 Which patients should be referred for an osteotomy?

Patients require careful selection as this operation is demanding mentally and physically compared to a joint replacement. The results are not as good

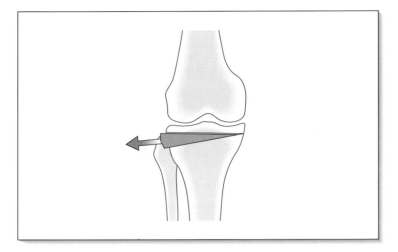

▲

BOX 11.2 Factors excluding an osteotomy

■ Severe patellofemoral disease
■ Severe malalignment
■ Mentally or physically frail patients
■ Poor 'activity age'
■ Severely advanced joint disease
■ Advanced obesity

---

as for joint replacements (*see Q. 11.18*); also, healing takes longer with a consequent longer stay in hospital. The operation should be reserved for patients who have severe knee pain and high activity demands, such as a farmer who wishes to continue farming where there is high impact and high activity, or when hobbies are very active (e.g. an enthusiastic skier or hill walker). In essence, the patient will have an activity age of 60 or less.

11.18 Are there factors that exclude an osteotomy?

Yes. Obviously all factors are relative, but a number of exclusion factors can be identified (*see Box 11.2*).

Results of osteotomy vary much more than those for joint replacements and even optimal candidates may quickly develop recurrence of pain and loss of function. Figures for the beneficial effects of osteotomy are around 90% at 1 year, falling to 70% at 5 years; by 10 years they have fallen to 30%. Importantly, an osteotomy can be converted to an arthroplasty.

11.19 Who should be offered a unicompartmental (unicondylar) knee replacement?

The patients who fit the criteria for this operation will have medial or lateral compartment disease with moderate or severe pain and functional impairment. Best results are obtained if there is minimal patellofemoral disease, a stable knee and little malalignment.

This operation used to have a very limited place and was not favoured by surgeons, probably because the figures for loosening are about twice as high as for total knee replacement. Revision rates are therefore much higher, but a revision of a failed unicompartmental implant is less complex than for a total knee replacement. For this reason, improved devices are being reconsidered for persons with an activity age of 60 or less.

The other group of patients who are being reconsidered for this operation are the more elderly and frail as the operation is less demanding on them both mentally and physically. The patient spends less time in the operating theatre and in the hospital ward. There is less likelihood of disorientation and a greater chance of quicker mobilization and return to independence.

11.20 What is an arthrodesis and for which joints is it useful?

This is an operation to fix the bones across a joint. The outcome will be a strong lever. An arthrodesis may be used to stabilize a failed knee or hip arthroplasty. A patient may request information as to the alternatives and consequences of a completely failed or infected arthroplasty (knee or hip) before they agree to a specific joint replacement; an arthrodesis is one alternative. It is a relatively simple operation giving a pain-free result and usually a better quality of life, provided that the other joints compensate for the loss of movement.

The carpometacarpal joint of the thumb rarely requires an arthrodesis for OA, but this will give a pain-free joint with only limited loss of dexterity.

A 'natural arthrodesis' may be seen in patients with RA, especially across wrist joints, giving them a strong 'lever' and improved finger use.

11.21 What information should be given to a patient postoperatively?

Patient management is on-going. Patient education starts at the time of referral. In this way, a patient understands what will happen next and can be given reassurance if necessary. A well-informed patient helps the overall outcome of operations (*see Qs 11.22 and 11.23*).

11.22 What advice should be given to patients and carers to improve surgical outcomes?

Points to remember for patients and carers:

- Attainable goals for the patient should be realistic.
- The patient must fully understand the purpose and goals of his or her exercise regime.
- The patient must have the ability to undertake these exercises.
- Patients will require reassurance and encouragement. Many patients discontinue the exercises and do not gain full benefit from their operation.
- Social support for recovery at home must be adequate. Patients and carers will need advice on what to do, what not to do, how to cope and when to seek help. Many hospitals have a helpline to advise patients, carers and doctors.
- Any potential problems and pitfalls, both common and specific, should be explained to the patient and carer.
- The anticipated time scale of progression must be explained; for example, it is important to realize that physical improvements can continue for up to 1–2 years.
- The joint may become painful and swollen. If this happens, apply ice and temporarily decrease the exercise regime. Remember that prolonged immobilization increases the risk of postoperative complications. This applies especially to muscle atrophy, which will lead to a decreased range of movements and may thereby impede overall attainment.

11.23 How could postoperative management and co-operation be improved?

By continuing to improve communications between doctors, patients and carers. This may be facilitated by using a locally designed referral form (*see Fig. 11.4*). The form should include information about physiotherapy, range of movement, walking aids, driving and expected functional gain. It should contain a helpline number.

11.24 Do hip arthroplasties do better than knee arthroplasties?

The outcomes are probably the same. Historically, the public and doctors have considered that knee arthroplasties do not achieve the quality results of hip arthroplasties. We have long memories that result in concepts being perpetuated for generations. The original hinged knee joints were poor, but

Patient name (last name, first name) .... Birth date (yy-mm-dd) ....
Patient address, phone ....
Date of referral .... Referring doctor .... Practice ....
....

Patient data   Male ☐   Female ☐   Age ....

Operation   Date of operation .... Length of hospital stay .... days

Arthroscopy   ☐
Osteotomy   ☐
Unicompartmental arthroplasty ☐
Bi/tricompartmental arthroplasty ☐
Other type of surgery   ☐   Specify ....
                                                     ....

Postoperative complications   infection ☐ deep vein thrombosis ☐ PE ☐
                                        other   ☐ Specify ....
                                                      ....

Rehabilitation and follow-up suggested

Specific rehabilitation   Yes ☐ No ☐ Time .... weeks
Physiotherapy   Yes ☐ No ☐ Time .... weeks
Use of walking aid   Yes ☐ No ☐ Time .... weeks
Wound treatment   Yes ☐ No ☐ Specify ....
                                                   ....
                                            Time .... weeks
Calf/knee swelling treatment   Yes ☐ No ☐ Specify ....
                                                   ....
                                            Time .... weeks
Anti-thrombotic therapy   Yes ☐ No ☐ Specify ....
                                                   ....
                                            Time .... weeks

Patient activity and expected outcome of surgery

Expected range of movement   .... degrees
Possible minor complications   pain ☐ for .... weeks   swelling ☐ for ....weeks
Full weight bearing expected   now ☐ after .... weeks
Patient may drive car   now ☐ after .... weeks
Expected functional gain at 6 months ....
....

Patient must **NOT** do impact sports or heavy work

General information
Patient must be reminded that after arthroplasty the knee is expected to be stable
and pain free, but that the knee will not be a normal knee

Helpline phone number ....

▲

Fig. 11.4 Example of a postoperative referral form. From Hosie G, Dickson J 2000
Managing osteoarthritis in primary care (Blackwell Science) with permission.

things have changed. The recent 5-year statistics for both knees and hips are excellent; in fact, the knee survival figures are better than those for hips.

The other misconception is based around the different rehabilitation stages of the two procedures (*see Q. 11.25*).

11.25 Why do knee arthroplasties appear to do less well than hips?

Overall there is little difference, although in fact knees do better (*see Q. 11.24*). It is during the rehabilitation stage that false assumptions are made.

After hip arthroplasties patients are mobilized rapidly and are virtually pain-free within 24 h; in some hospital programmes patients are discharged at this stage.

In marked contrast, the rehabilitation for knee arthroplasties is much longer. The pain can be severe during the days after the operation and will fluctuate over the following weeks and months. Despite this, the 1-year results are excellent.

This initial negative comparison must be explained to patients otherwise they, and their friends and carers, will have unrealistic expectations, which can lead to depression and slow recovery. If the referring doctor explains initially that the road to recovery is a little steeper and more painful, it will help in reducing the risk of postoperative complications. Patients often need reassurance postoperatively in order to exercise and mobilize with confidence, which in turn helps to keep pain to a minimum and leads to a speedy recovery.

11.26 What options are there for young patients with severe OA of the hip or knee?

The major problem in young patients is that they are more active and are therefore more likely to wear out replacement joints and so require further joint replacements. On the other hand, they have good muscles that will protect the joint, so this group of patients often have good joint replacement survival rates.

Orthopaedic surgeons may try to re-align stresses (e.g. perform arthroplasties). Earlier in the disease process the use of hyaluronans may be considered. For hips, these injections are usually performed using ultrasound for guidance.

The greatest advance has been in the design, engineering and materials used in replacement joints. It is now possible to make metal-on-metal and similar prostheses which show virtually no signs of wear and tear. These modern joints are very expensive and it is too early, as yet, to confirm the expected survival rates.

11.27 What surgical options are there for active older patients with severe knee OA?

Basically, the options are an osteotomy or a modern unicompartmental arthroplasty (*see Qs 11.18 and 11.19*).

Prognosis

12

12.1 What happens to patients with OA?

Most patients will lead an active life hardly affected by their joint disease. Around 10% of patients with OA will have disease that will seriously affect their quality of life. Some patients from this 10% will require arthroplasty. The revision rates for arthroplasty for knee and hip are rising, but in essence they are around 1 per 1000 for both knee and hip in patients aged over 65.

12.2 Will OA become as severe as RA?

This is most unlikely as OA and RA (rheumatoid arthritis) are two different forms of arthritis. Patients with RA tend to have a much more aggressive type of disease, and rapid deterioration in function, so that disability is severe from early in the course of the disease. OA has a slower progression, usually moving forward in flares of pain and disability that last a few days to a few weeks, then settles. Sometimes patients have no more flares and only have mild disability and minor loss of function. The vast majority of patients will not be disabled by their arthritis (*see Q. 12.1*).

12.3 Can OA improve?

Yes. We are biological beings, meaning that there is always repair as well as destruction occurring and these are usually in balance (*see Fig. 12.1*). The concept is that, in OA, more destruction is taking place than repair. Mechanical and physical interventions are aimed at decreasing/limiting destruction and allowing repair to take place. In many patients this happens naturally, but in OA knees, for example, quadriceps exercises and the use of shock-absorbing shoes or insoles are expected to aid natural repair.

12.4 If one hip is replaced, will the other large joints require replacement too?

OA tends to affect the dominant side most commonly, and patients very often have only one affected large joint (i.e. one knee or one hip). There is another group of patients who appear to have more generalized disease with multiple joints affected. This smaller group of patients, who are seen in clinics on more occasions, may well require four arthroplasties.

12.5 Is it possible to replace thumb joints?

Yes, but a better operation is an arthrodesis (*see Q. 11.20*).

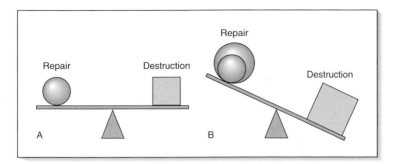

▲

Fig. 12.1 Diagram to illustrate the balance between repair and destruction of tissue in a normal joint (a) and the effect of OA on this balance (b). In OA, both destruction and repair processes speed up, but the effect of destruction is greater. From Hosie G, Dickson J 2000 Managing osteoarthritis in primary care (Blackwell Science) with permission.

12.6   Do thumb joint replacements last?

No (*see Q. 11.20*).

12.7   Does the pain in OA joints continue to increase?

Increasing pain is a 'red flag'. Trauma, infection and cancer must be considered. Pain of OA may be severe but it rarely continues to increase unless the femoral head is collapsing. Bone-on-bone gives the worst pain in OA, giving the triad 'can't sleep, can't walk, can't work'.

12.8   Does joint replacement always stop the joint pain?

Yes, with the proviso that patients who have had to wait longer for operation are more likely to develop the syndrome of chronic pain. In these patients some amount of chronic pain may become the diagnosis and this will need managing. (Readers are referred to the Arthritis Research Campaign *Rheumatic Disease: In Practice* series nos 9 and 10, details of which can be found on the ARC website; *see Appendix 3*.)

12.9   Do pain management strategies work in the long term?

Yes, but pain, especially chronic pain and its consequences on patients' quality of life and disability, will fluctuate over time.

12.10   Will complementary therapy adversely affect the prognosis for OA?

No. Complementary therapies may well relieve patients' anxieties and allow a better quality of life, which will probably lead to increased mobility. This in turn will lead to greater muscle strength and it is the muscles that protect the joints.

12.11 Will a lateral heel wedge reduce the likelihood of requiring a total knee replacement?

In theory, wedges are used to take the load off the most affected compartment of the knee. The evidence to give a Yes or No answer is not yet available. There is work that shows that patients decrease the use of NSAIDs if heel wedges are used. X-ray changes have not been seen but it is possible that the trials were not conducted for a long enough time frame (*see Q. 5.12*).

PQ PATIENT QUESTIONS

12.12 What can I do to improve the prognosis (long-term outcome) of my OA?

■ Believe that OA will not cause severe disability.
■ Use shock-absorbing shoes/insoles (e.g. trainers, Ecco or Hotter shoes, sorbothane insoles).
■ Use your joints sensibly to maintain or build up your muscles as these protect your joints. Quadriceps exercises will help knee OA.
■ If you have OA hand, use gloves when possible, so that you grip well but do not grip too hard.
■ Use a walking stick in the opposite hand if you have hip or knee OA. It will take 25% of the weight off the painful joint.
■ Lose weight if you are overweight (i.e. by about 14 lb or 8 kg), as a loss of 10% of your body weight can relieve pain by up to 50%.

12.13 I've had one large joint replacement. Is it inevitable that I will need more joint replacements?

No. Many patients only require one. Some people do require multiple replacements and this may be discussed when you first see the orthopaedic surgeon. If you have one badly affected joint other joints will also often be affected (*see Q. 12.4*).

12.14 I was in my 50s when I had my hip/knee replaced. How do I look after this one to reduce the likelihood of requiring a revision?

The larger the muscles around a joint the more these muscles protect the joint. Have a decent quality of life by keeping up your hobbies, especially walking and golf. Remember to wear shock-absorbing shoes and insoles and do not become obese. If you are overweight, go on a diet.

12.15 My hands have lots of lumps and bumps on them. Will I lose the use of them when I'm older?

No. This is very unlikely. OA of the hands causes some loss of function but nothing like the loss of function experienced in RA (rheumatoid arthritis). A simple analogy is to consider that OA hands may cause you to drop one cup a week whereas RA will cause the breakage of two daily.

12.16 If I take my NSAIDs/COX-2 inhibitors regularly will they stop my arthritis from getting worse?

These drugs have not been shown to have an effect on the OA disease process, but if they relieve the pain and make you more mobile because you have greater use of your joints and muscles then this may protect you.

12.17 I have arthritis, as did my mother. She needed a new hip, will I?

Genes have a lot to answer for. It is possible that you may require a new hip but by using joint protection (*see Qs 12.1 and 12.2*) this may be delayed or even prevented.

12.18 Are there any foods or diets that will have an effect on my arthritis in the long term?

Evidence on diets for any form of arthritis is very difficult to find. For advice on glucosamine and similar products see Ch. 5 and Ch. 10 (*Q. 10.17*).

The advice concerning polyunsaturated fatty acids (fish oils, etc.) is scanty and there is no hard evidence for their use in OA to date. There is evidence that, when large quantities of fish oils are taken, the immune system responses are suppressed, allowing the NSAID/COX-2 inhibitor dosage to be reduced.

Referral strategies

13

13.1 Which patients should be referred to an orthopaedic surgeon?

The ideal orthopaedic patient is one who needs an operation and wants to be operated upon.

Historically, orthopaedic services have been used as a sorting house for primary care musculoskeletal patients. This has led to long waiting times for outpatient clinics, possibly poor medical management and, at worst, inappropriate surgical procedures. With the expansion of primary care trusts and the development of musculoskeletal services, this situation is likely to change. There will be more physiotherapists who will often be qualified to perform injections and supply simple off-the-shelf appliances.

Primary care will also have more access to specialist investigations so that more appropriate and 'worked-up' patients will be referred to orthopaedic surgeons (*see Q. 13.3 and Ch. 11*).

13.2 Which patients should be referred to a rheumatologist?

These days, rheumatologists wish to see patients who have, or may have, inflammatory arthritis. To diagnose these problems early is not easy. Some units have introduced early arthritis clinics where there is virtually open access for patients to be screened and investigated. The percentage of inflammatory arthritis is around 50% in these clinics. The other 50% is made up of reactive arthritis, fibromyalgia and other diagnoses.

13.3 When do patients require referral for X-rays?

An X-ray should only be taken when the result will influence a management change or if the diagnosis is uncertain. In essence, this often means that the patient requires a surgical opinion. Many general practitioners will X-ray patients at all 'stages' of OA and Bedson et al (2002) have shown that the X-ray report will influence management decisions.

Patients who complain of anterior knee pain will often have clinically relatively normal-looking knees and the weight-bearing X-rays may be reported as 'normal'. These patients require skyline views to look at the patellofemoral compartment of the joint.

13.4 Do patients with OA require referral for DEXA scans?

No. A DEXA (dual-energy X-ray absorption) scan will not be helpful for osteoarthritis. There is a negative association between osteoporosis and OA (*see Q. 1.12*).

13.5 When should physiotherapy be requested?

Physiotherapy should play a major role in the modern management of OA. Physiotherapists are particularly good at patient education and reassurance and are therefore extremely valuable members of the primary care team. This role must be encouraged as it plays a large part in pain relief and so improves the patient's quality of life. The knee joint causes the greatest disability and the physiotherapist's role is invaluable for advice about exercise, quadriceps strengthening, improving mobility, shock-absorbing footwear, as well as education and confidence-building.

13.6 Which patients benefit from occupational therapy advice?

It is probable that all patients could benefit, but this is not a practical proposition. Occupational help should be offered to patients who are at greatest need. These patients are usually those who are house-bound or very dependent on others, especially those who for medical or personal reasons are unable to have joint replacements. Patients with severe hand OA, especially if there is an inflammatory component to the disease, will definitely benefit from occupational therapy advice and help.

13.7 When should help from pain management specialists be requested?

Chronic pain is difficult to manage and all avenues of help should be explored. Staff with expertise in cognitive therapy are a great asset. Physiotherapists and occupational therapists should be consulted; unfortunately, few primary care teams have access to psychologists. Patients who find it difficult to cope with life are the ones in greatest need of help. These patients require referral to a pain management specialist, but the waiting list is usually extensive. A long-term solution may lie in persuading primary care trusts to fund community mini-teams. (For further help and advice, see the Arthritis Research Campaign *Rheumatic Disease: In Practice* series nos 9–11, details of which can be found on the ARC website; *see Appendix 3*.)

13.8 Is a referral to a sports physiotherapist useful for patients with OA?

People with arthritis are encouraged to partake in sporting activities and will benefit from specialist advice. A sports physiotherapist is experienced in giving quality advice to sporting enthusiasts of all ages, whether they have arthritis, other disabilities or are fit. This is especially valuable to people over 50 who wish to take exercise, as our bodies become less resilient with age.

13.9 When is a podiatrist of use for patients with OA?

Podiatrists are experts in all things to do with feet, and their knowledge of bio-engineering may also help with problems relating to knees and hips. For an opinion about feet, a referral to a podiatrist should be considered before referral to an orthopaedic surgeon. Appropriate advice and the use of orthotics such as insoles should be considered before operative procedures.

13.10 What orthotic help is useful?

Shock-absorbing shoes are advisable for all patients with large joint OA. Advice about insoles and other orthotics can be obtained from appliance officers and podiatrists.

13.11 Which is the most important: physiotherapy referral before operation for arthroplasty or physiotherapy referral after operation for arthroplasty?

Both. If muscle strength can be maintained before an arthroplasty then the results will be improved. The greater the muscle strength, the better quality of life is likely to be. The proof of this is comes from recent studies in Sweden which show that the older the patient and the longer the wait for hip arthroplasty, the poorer the final result. This probably applies to knees also. Obtaining physiotherapy before operation is probably a luxury in the NHS, but patients should be encouraged to continue with as much activity as possible and encouraged to swim.

Postoperative physiotherapy is essential in order that patients can obtain maximum benefit from an expensive operation. It is also important to encourage patients to continue with these exercises for at least a year postoperatively; this can often be done by regular contact (phone calls) or patient group therapy/exercise sessions.

13.12 Patients awaiting a knee or hip replacement often have severe pain. What help is available?

On a practical basis, it is impossible to refer these patients to a pain clinic as there is usually such a long waiting list. It is worthwhile referring to a practitioner who gives injections. Patients awaiting hip arthroplasty will often have a trochanteric bursitis and will benefit from an appropriately placed steroid/lidocaine (lignocaine) injection. Similarly, with knee pain, lidocaine with or without steroid, placed in the area of the anserine bursa will greatly relieve a patient's suffering. These injections may need to be repeated depending on the length of the orthopaedic waiting list.

13.13 Which patients require pre-operative assessment?

All patients should be assessed by the pre-operative assessment team.

13.14 How can we reduce the number of referrals to orthopaedic surgeons?

Many primary care trusts and hospital departments are re-evaluating referral pathways. Historically, most musculoskeletal problems were referred to orthopaedic surgeons. This is at last being questioned, as their primary training is in surgical answers to problems rather than to take a medical approach. It is probable that over 80% of these referrals could be managed medically, and referral pathways through physiotherapy and podiatry are being instigated. Some personnel in these departments have additional qualifications, such as a diploma in injection techniques. These initiatives should decrease waiting times for patients and even reduce the number of operations, but this approach will require new concepts of delivery of care and teams working together for the benefit of the patients.

PQ PATIENT QUESTIONS

13.15 How can I be referred to the local self-help group?

It is always worthwhile asking the receptionist or looking for leaflets from Arthritis Care in your doctor's surgery. Otherwise try your local library, the local arthritis charity shop, a telephone directory, or enquire at the hospital rheumatology department. Literature from Arthritis Care, usually available at the doctor's surgery, will give phone numbers and website details that will give you the contact details of your nearest self-help group (*see Appendix 3*).

13.16 When should I ask for another opinion?

You should not be afraid to ask for a second opinion or to discuss this option with your doctor. Most doctors are quite happy to refer a patient, especially if there are still unanswered questions and the patient is still having problems. If new diagnoses or answers are found, then things can move forward; if not, then at least the patient feels that nothing is being missed and the GP's relationship with the patient is reinforced.

If you are unhappy with a diagnosis, or the lack of one, then discuss the situation with your GP and decide whether or not you would like a further opinion.

13.17 Why is there such a long wait for pain clinics?

Chronic pain and its management frequently present problems. There are not enough pain clinics to meet the demand. It is hoped that, in future, primary care trusts may commission similar clinics run from a primary care base. There are some good articles about chronic pain and disability on the ARC website ('In Practice' section; *see Appendix 3*).

13.18 Can I be referred for acupuncture for my hip/knee pain?

Yes. Many physiotherapists and some GPs are trained in acupuncture techniques. You may be referred to a physiotherapist working at your doctor's surgery, in the community or at a hospital.

APPENDIX 1: WOMAC (WESTERN ONTARIO AND MCMASTER) OSTEOARTHRITIS INDEX

This is a three-dimensional, self-administered measure specific to OA, looking at pain, stiffness and physical function in OA of hip or knee (Bellamy et al 1988). The assessment formats are either a visual analogue scale or a Likert scale (*Fig. A.1*). There are 24 questions: five on pain, two on stiffness and 17 on physical function.

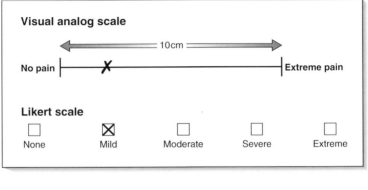

▲

Fig. A.1 WOMAC visual analogue and Likert scales From Bellamy et al 1998 with permission.

APPENDIX 2: LEQUESNE ALGOFUNCTIONAL INDICES

There are two indices, one for hip and one for knee, looking at pain, maximum distance walked and activities of daily living. These indices are more difficult for patients to self-administer than the WOMAC and may require an interviewer. Questions are asked and points allocated according to the patient's reply (a high score indicates greater severity).

For example, for pain or discomfort during nocturnal bed rest:

- ■ None or insignificant: 0
- ■ Only on movement or in certain positions: 1
- ■ With no movement: 2.

APPENDIX 3
Useful addresses and websites

USEFUL ADDRESSES

BRITISH SOCIETY FOR RHEUMATOLOGY
41 Eagle Street
London WC1R 4TL
Tel: 020 7242 3313
Fax: 020 7242 3277
http://www.rheumatology.org.uk

ARTHRITIS CARE
18 Stephenson Way
London NW1 2HD
Tel: 020 7380 6500
Fax: 020 7380 6505
http://www.arthritiscare.org.uk

ARTHRITIS RESEARCH CAMPAIGN
Copeman House
St Mary's Gate
Chesterfield S41 7TD
Tel: 01246 558033
Fax: 01246 558007
http://www.arc.org.uk

EUROPEAN LEAGUE AGAINST ARTHRITIS (EULAR)
Eular Executive Secretariat
Witikonerstrasse 15
Zurich
Switzerland
Tel: 0041 1383 9690
Fax: 0041 1383 9810
http://www.eular.org

PRIMARY CARE RHEUMATOLOGY SOCIETY
PO Box 42
Northallerton DL7 8YG
Tel: 01609 774 794
Fax: 01609 774 726
http://www.pcrsociety.com

POSTGRADUATE DIPLOMA IN PRIMARY CARE RHEUMATOLOGY (PCR)
Department of Medicine Sciences
University of Bath
Bath BA2 7AY
Tel: 01225 383611
Fax: 01225 383833
http://www.bath.ac.uk/med-sci/PCR.htm

AMERICAN COLLEGE OF RHEUMATOLOGY
1800 Century Place
Suite 250
Atlanta, GA 30345
USA
Tel: 001 404 633 3777
Fax: 001 404 633 1870
http://www.rheumatology.org

USEFUL WEBSITES
Move (making osteoarthritis matter)
http://www.move.uk.net
Bandolier
http://www.jr2.ox.ac.uk/bandolier
Oxford Pain Research
http://www.jr2.ox.ac.uk/bandolier/painres/PRintro.html
Cochrane Collaboration
http://www.cochrane.org
NHS Centre for Reviews and Dissemination, University of York
http://www.york.ac.uk/inst/crd/welcome.htm
Evidence Based Healthcare Resources
http://www.northglashealthinfo.org.uk

ESPECIALLY FOR SEARCHING
PubMed (database which includes citations not yet on MEDLINE)
http://www.ncbi.nih.gov/PubMed
Biomednet (databases include 'evaluated' MEDLINE)
http://www.bmn.com
BIDS (UK non-profit-making database providers; home of EMBASE)
http://www.bids.ac.uk
CISCOM (centralized information service for complementary medicine)
http://www.rccm.org.uk/ciscom
OMNI (Organising Medical Networked Information; provides search
engine for various websites and access to MEDLINE)
http://www.omni.ac.uk

REFERENCES AND FURTHER READING

Chapter 1

Doherty M, Lanyon P, Hosie G 2001 Osteoarthritis of the knee and hip. Rheumatic disease: in practice no 4. Arthritis Research Campaign

Engel A 1968 Osteoarthritis and body measurements. National Center for Health Statistics, Rockville, MD

Felson DT, Naimark A, Anderson J et al 1987 The prevalence of knee osteoarthritis in the elderly. Arthritis and Rheumatism 30:914–918

Felson DT, Zhang Y, Anthony JM et al 1992 Weight loss reduces the risk for symptomatic knee osteoarthritis in women. Annals of Internal Medicine 116:535–539

Hannan MT, Felson DT, Anderson JJ et al 1990 Estrogen use and radiographic osteoarthritis of the knee in women. Arthritis and Rheumatism 33:525–532

Nevitt MC, Cummings SR, Lane NE et al 1994 Current use of oral estrogen is associated with a decreased prevalence of radiographic hip OA in elderly white women. Arthritis and Rheumatism 37(suppl):S212

Peat G, McCarney R, Croft P 2001 Knee pain and osteoarthritis in older adults: a review of community burden and current use of primary health care. Annals of the Rheumatic Diseases 60:91–97

Chapter 2

Hochberg MC, Altman RD, Brandt KD et al 1995 Guidelines for the medical management of osteoarthritis. Part 1: Osteoarthritis of the hip. Part 2: Osteoarthritis of the knee. Arthritis and Rheumatism 38(11):1541–1546

Chapter 5

Cushnaghan J, McCarthy C, Dieppe P 1994 Taping the patella medially: a new treatment for osteoarthritis of the knee joint? BMJ 308:753–755

Ezzo J, Hadhazy V, Birch S et al 2001 Acupuncture for osteoarthritis of the knee: a systematic review. Arthritis and Rheumatism 44:819–825

Hurley MV, Scott DL 1998 Improvements in quadriceps sensorimotor function and disability of patients with knee osteoarthritis following a clinically practicable exercise regime. British Journal of Rheumatology 37:1181–1187

Long L, Ernst E 2001 Homeopathic remedies for the treatment of osteoarthritis: a systematic review. British Homeopathy Journal 90(3):175–176

Long L, Soeken K, Ernst E 2001 Herbal medicines for the treatment of osteoarthritis: a systematic review. Rheumatology 40:779–793

Sutton AJ, Muir KR, Mockett S et al 2001 A case controlled study to investigate the relationship between low and moderate levels of physical activity and osteoarthritis of the knee using data collected as part of the Allied Dunbar National Fitness Survey. Annals of the Rheumatic Diseases 60:756–769

Chapter 6

Hochberg MC, Altman RD, Brandt KD et al 1995 Guidelines for the medical management of osteoarthritis. Part 1: Osteoarthritis of the hip. Part 2: Osteoarthritis of the knee. Arthritis and Rheumatism 38(11):1541–1546

Moore RA, Tramer MR, Carroll D et al 1998 Review. Topical non-steroidal anti-inflammatory drugs are effective and safe for pain. BMJ 316:333–338

Chapter 8

Bombardier C, Laine L, Reicin A et al 2000 Comparison of upper gastro-intestinal toxicity of rofecoxib and naproxen in patients with rheumatoid arthritis. VIGOR study group. New England Journal of Medicine 343:1520–1528

Dieppe P, Cushnaghan J, Jasani MK et al 1993 A two year, placebo-controlled trial of non-steroidal anti-inflammatory therapy in osteoarthritis of the knee joint. British Journal of Rheumatology 32:595–600

Fries JF, Spitz PW, Williams CA et al 1990 A toxicity index for comparison of side effects among different drugs. Arthritis and Rheumatism 33:121–130

Hochberg MC, Altman RD, Brandt KD et al 1995 Guidelines for the medical management of osteoarthritis. Part 1: Osteoarthritis of the hip. Part 2: Osteoarthritis of the knee. Arthritis and Rheumatism 38(11):1541–1546

Labenz J, Blum AL, Bolton WW et al 2002 Primary prevention of diclofenac associated ulcers and dyspepsia by omeprazole or triple therapy in Helicobacter pylori positive patients: a randomized, double blind, placebo controlled clinical trial. Gut 51:329–335

MacDonald TM, Morant SV, Robinson GC et al 1997 Association of upper gastrointestinal toxicity of non-steroidal anti-inflammatory drugs with continued exposure: cohort study. BMJ 315:1333–1337

National Institute for Clinical Excellence 2001 Guidance on the use of cyclooxygenase (COX) II selective inhibitors, celecoxib, rofecoxib, meloxicam and etodolac, for osteoarthritis and rheumatoid arthritis. NICE

Silverstein FE, Faich G, Goldstein JL et al 2000 Gastrointestinal toxicity with celecoxib vs nonsteroidal anti-inflammatory drugs for osteoarthritis and rheumatoid arthritis: the CLASS study: a randomised controlled trial. Celecoxib Long-term Arthritis Safety Study. JAMA 284:1247–1255

Tramer MR, Moore RA, Reynolds DJM et al 2000 Qualitative estimation of rare adverse events which follow a biological progression: a new model applied to chronic NSAID use. Pain 85:169–182

Chapter 9

Adebajo A, Nash P, Hazleman B 1990 A prospective double-blind dummy-placebo-controlled study comparing triamcinolone hexacetonide injection with oral diclofenac in patients with rotator cuff tendonitis. Journal of Rheumatology 17:1207–1210

Berry H, Fernandes L, Bloom B et al 1980 Clinical study comparing acupuncture, physiotherapy, injection and oral anti-inflammatory therapy in the shoulder. Current Medical Research Opinion 7:121–126

Jones A, Regan M, Ledingham J et al 1993 Importance of placement of intra-articular steroid injections. BMJ 307:1329–1330

Petri M, Dobrow R, Neiman R et al 1987 Randomized double-blind placebo-controlled study of the treatment of the painful shoulder. Arthritis and Rheumatism 30:1040–1045

Rizk T, Pinals T, Talaiver A 1991 Corticosteroid injections in adhesive capulitis: investigation of their value and site. Archives of Physical Medicine 72:70–72

Seror P, Pluvinage P, Lecoq d'Andre F et al 1999 Frequency of sepsis after local corticosteroid injection (an inquiry on 1160000 injections in rheumatological private practice in France). Rheumatology 38:1272–1274

Vecchio PC, Hazleman BL, King RH 1993 A double blind trial comparing subacromial methylprednisolone and lignocaine in acute rotator cuff tendonitis. British Journal of Rheumatology 32:743–745

Chapter 10

Hughes R, Carr A 2002 A randomised, double-blind, placebo-controlled trial of glucosamine sulphate as an analgesic in osteoarthritis of the knee. Rheumatology 41:279–284

McAlindon TE, LaValley MP, Gulin JP et al 2000 Glucosamine and chondroitin for treatment of osteoarthritis: a systematic quality assessment and meta-analysis. JAMA 283:1469–1475

Reginster JY, Deroisy R, Rovati LC et al 2001 Long term effects of glucosamine sulphate on osteoarthritis progression: a randomised, placebo-controlled clinical trial. Lancet 357:251–256

Chapter 11

Fortin PR, Clarke AD, Joseph L et al 1999 Outcomes of total hip and knee replacements. Pre-operative functional status predicts outcomes at six months after surgery. Arthritis and Rheumatism 42:1722–1728

Moseley JB, O'Malley K, Petersen NJ et al 2002 A controlled trial of arthroscopic surgery for osteoarthritis of the knee. New England Journal of Medicine 347:81–88

Negret P, Donnell ST, Dejour H 1994 Osteoarthritis of the knee following meniscectomy. British Journal of Rheumatology 33:367–368

Nilsdotter AK, Petersson IF, Roos EM et al 2002 Predictors of unsatisfactory patient-relevant outcome after total hip replacements for osteoarthritis. Annals of the Rheumatic Diseases 61(suppl 1):40

Roos H, Lauren M, Roos E et al 1998 Risk factors and osteoarthrosis after menisectomy. Arthritis and Rheumatism 41(suppl 9):abstract 326

Chapter 13

Bedson J, Jordan K, Croft PR 2002 The primary care management of chronic knee pain in the elderly. Rheumatology 41(suppl 1):poster 338

Appendix 1

Bellamy N, Buchanan WW, Goldsmith CH et al 1988 Validation study of WOMAC: a health status instrument for measuring clinically important patient relevant outcomes to antirheumatic drug therapy in patients with osteoarthritis of the hip or knee. Journal of Rheumatology 15:1833–1840

Appendix 2

Lequesne MG, Mery C, Samson M et al 1987 Indexes of severity for osteoarthritis of the hip and knee. Validation: value in comparison with other assessment tests. Scandinavian Journal of Rheumatology Supplement 65:85–89

Useful journal references

Barlow JH, Turner AP, Wright CC 1998 Long term outcomes of an arthritis self-management programme. Journal of Rheumatology 37:1315–1319

Dieppe P, Basler HD, Chard J et al 1999 Knee replacement surgery for osteoarthritis: effectiveness, practice variations, indications and possible determinants of utilization. Rheumatology 38:73–83

Eccles M, Freemantle N, Mason J et al 1998 North of England evidence based guideline development project: summary guideline for non-steroidal anti-inflammatory drugs versus basic analgesia in treating the pain of degenerative arthritis. BMJ 317:526–536

Felson DT, Zhang Y 1998 An update on the epidemiology of knee and hip osteoarthritis with a view to prevention. Arthritis and Rheumatism 41(8):1343–1355

Lorig KR, Mazonson PD, Holman HR 1993 Evidence suggesting that health education for self-management in patients with chronic arthritis has sustained health benefits while reducing health care costs. Arthritis and Rheumatism 36(4):439–446

Moore A, Phillips CJ 1999 Cost of NSAID

adverse effects to the UK National Health Service. Journal of Medical Economics 2:45–55

Scott DL 1993 Guidelines for the diagnosis, investigation and management of osteoarthritis of the hip and knee. Report of a joint working group of the British Society for Rheumatology and the Research Unit of the Royal College of Physicians. Journal of the Royal College of Physicians of London 27(4)

Reference books

Brandt KD, Doherty ML. Lohmander LS (eds) 1998 Osteoarthritis. Oxford University Press (ISBN 0-19-262735-X)

Hosie G, Field M 2002 Shared care in rheumatology. Martin Dunitz (ISBN 1-901865-10-X)

Klippel J, Dieppe P 1998 Rheumatology. Mosby-Yearbook (Europe) (ISBN 07234 2405 5)

Klippel J, Dieppe P, Ferri FF 1999 Primary care rheumatology. Mosby (ISBN 07234-3143-4)

Silver T 1999 Joint and soft tissue injection, 2nd edn. Radcliffe Medical Press (ISBN 1-85775-341-0)

Snaith M 1996 ABC of rheumatology. BMJ Publishing Group (ISBN 0-7279-0997-5)

University of Bath and Primary Care Rheumatology Society 1995 Diploma of primary care rheumatology by distance learning. Distance Learning Unit, University of Bath

LIST OF PATIENT QUESTIONS

INDEX

Numbers in **bold** refer to figures and tables.

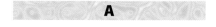

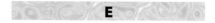
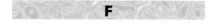
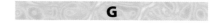

I

J

K

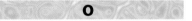

N

O

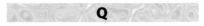

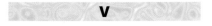

U

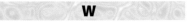

V

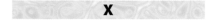

W

X

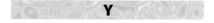

Y